Beginning Wildlife Rehab

Beginning Wildlife Rehab

✦

Things to Consider Before Becoming a Licensed Colorado Wildlife Rehabilitator

Donna J. Ralph

iUniverse, Inc.
New York Lincoln Shanghai

Beginning Wildlife Rehab
Things to Consider Before Becoming a Licensed Colorado Wildlife Rehabilitator

iUniverse books may be ordered through booksellers or by contacting:

iUniverse
2021 Pine Lake Road, Suite 100
Lincoln, NE 68512
www.iuniverse.com
1-800-Authors (1-800-288-4677)

Because of the dynamic nature of the Internet, any Web addresses or links contained in this book may have changed since publication and may no longer be valid.

The views expressed in this work are solely those of the author and do not necessarily reflect the views of the publisher, and the publisher hereby disclaims any responsibility for them.

ISBN: 978-0-595-48334-1 (pbk)
ISBN: 978-0-595-60424-1 (ebk)

Printed in the United States of America

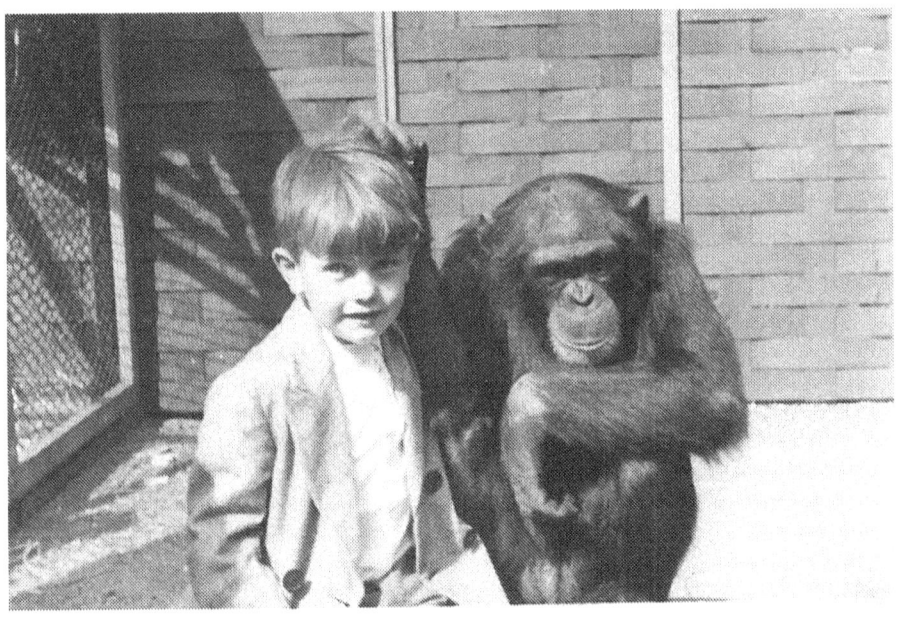

My Dad as a young boy at the London Zoo with his newfound animal pal.

This book is dedicated to everyone who respects and appreciates all animals, wild and otherwise. This book is dedicated to the caregivers of animals; the dedicated people who make enormous sacrifices to help those without voices.

Contents

FOREWORD

Let me start by saying this book is totally subjective and based only on my own personal experiences. I have no college education in the field of wildlife rehabilitation, or nonprofit or business management. I have learned, and am still learning, as I go. Everyone's experience will be unique to them. I started out as (and still am) a working person with no political or financial "connections" and have had nothing handed to me. I have worked very, very hard to get as far as I have, with a great distance still to go. When I started out as a rehabber I had gotten some good help and some not-so-good help. I've had to learn the hard way-by experience. I feel when you truly believe in something and if you are dedicated, you can accomplish something good.

I can tell you only of my personal experiences and the way the rules have applied to me in the State of Colorado. Laws vary from state to state and I truly recommend you familiarize yourself with the laws, and follow them very closely. The rules can and sometimes do change.

I write this book with the assumption that you'll be working out of your own home, as so many of us do, particularly in Colorado. If you'll be doing wildlife rehab in an out-of-the-house facility, lucky you-you get to clock out at the end of the day and might find that much of the information in this book doesn't apply to you.

I wrote this book because I hope that it will help you decide whether or not you want to become a licensed wildlife rehabilitator, and I hope that if you do decide to become licensed, that you will always keep the big picture and the best interest of the animals your Number 1 priority and never, ever forget your mission statement or allow yourself to get tripped up in your ego.

Sometimes I think that long-time rehabbers forget what it's like being new and starting out in this field. We aren't as patient and helpful as we could be to the "newbies." So this book is for the potential "newbie" rehabber. Hope you find it helpful.

I wrote this book because I've learned a few things along the way that were never addressed at conferences and meetings; thing I feel are important but sometimes difficult for people to talk about. I hope this book helps you. When I was new and starting out, I didn't find a good book for the beginner regarding the process; back then it seemed only the medical care books were available.

I write this book in the hopes that I am scaring you off, if you think of this work as a hobby or aren't fully committed to the work. Better I scare you off now than you find out the reality of this work as a trembling, sobbing heap on your living room floor with a house full of sick, hungry animals that you can't take care of.

Good luck!

IS WILDLIFE REHAB FOR YOU?

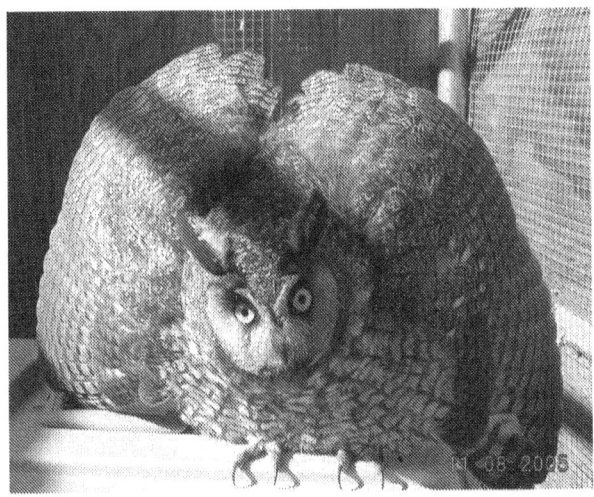

Long-eared owl

What is wildlife rehab? In Colorado, wildlife rehab is caring for sick, injured, and orphaned wild birds and mammals for the purpose of RELEASE. We do not keep them as pets, as this is illegal. Wildlife rehab is a way of life, not a hobby.

Only you can decide if wildlife rehabilitation is for you. If you have the luxuries of time and money, this might be something you would want to do. If you live paycheck to paycheck like I do, and have family, work, or other responsibilities, you might consider volunteering for a wildlife rehabilitator for a season-preferably the busy spring, summer, and fall baby seasons-to see if this is for you. Wildlife rehabilitation for the average, not well-connected individual that is a regular working person can be extremely challenging on many levels.

Why do you think you want to be a wildlife rehabilitator? Is it because you love animals and want to help? Do you think this work gives you some sort of prestige? (Not in my experience!) Do you want to help animals for their benefit or for yours?

You need to consider time. Do you have time? Will you be home-based? Because if you are, wildlife rehab could very well mean that you will give up a big part of your social and family life. These animals depend on YOU, and you must be committed to them. You'll miss dates, graduations, Super Bowl games, holidays, and other special occasions, unless you're lucky enough to have no animals during those times or are lucky enough to have another rehabber give you a break.

Consider your family and friends, and also remember wildlife rehab isn't something you're necessarily going to make a family event, as the animals need a stress-free environment and they don't get that in a house full of noisy people, pets, telephones, TV, etc. Only if you have a quiet indoor area away from the sights and sounds of people and pets can this work well.

Now back to your family. Will your kids and partner feel deprived of your time and attention while you tend to the animals, the ringing telephone, the running around, and the paperwork? How will they feel if you have to miss their football games/graduations/weddings, and so forth? Remember that this kind of work will require you to cancel plans at the very last minute if you get a call. Friends and family don't appreciate taking second place to your wildlife work. I know from experience that wildlife rehab can be the kiss of death to a social life!

About the money. This is a reality that you can't ignore. In Colorado we don't get paid to be wildlife rehabbers and we're not funded by anyone, either. We are solely responsible for all costs incurred; food, supplies, equipment, medical care, gas, and on and on. Whether you choose to care for only one animal at a time or a hundred, you have to consider their dietary, medical, and housing needs, not to mention the length of time they could be in rehab. Don't take animals you can't afford to feed! And don't rely on the individual showing up at your door with a shoebox full of baby birds to give you a donation, especially if you're not a non-profit. My experience over the years has been that the people most able to make a donation usually don't, and the people least likely to be able to donate are the ones that usually do. Some people will donate only if they get the tax write-off and you can't give them that if you're not an IRS nonprofit with the documentation to prove it.

When people bring an animal to our home-based facilities, they tend to think wildlife rehabilitation is a quaint little hobby. After all, if this were serious business, wouldn't there be a big glass and brick building, bustling with uniformed, paid staff? They don't understand that this isn't how it works in Colorado.

We spend a lot of our own paychecks doing this work and are always playing catch-up on our bills. Rehabbers can go into serious debt to do this work. Is becoming a nonprofit something you would consider?

Keep in mind that as a home-based rehabber, there will be a lot of wear and tear on your mind, your body, your car, your washer and dryer, your dishwasher, your microwave, your food processor….

You will probably need help to do wildlife rehab. Maybe you're lucky enough to have a partner that will help you with the day-to-day chores of wildlife rehab. If you provide care to more than a few birds or animals, I think you can count on the fact you will need help. I believe it is crucial that you have moral support from your spouse or partner to do this work. You will need a listening ear and a shoulder to cry upon. You will need someone that will let you vent without taking offense. Other rehabbers can be very helpful in this regard as well. Look for the ones that you can communicate well with; they are true treasures.

FOLLOWING THE RULES

I recommend maintaining a good working relationship with your wildlife agencies and wildlife officers, and keep the lines of communication very open. These are the people that can help you and these are also the people that can shut you down. Although wildlife officers and agencies tend to have more of a focus on law enforcement, they likely care just as much about wildlife as you do, otherwise they probably wouldn't be working in the wildlife field. Be honest and open with them, and let them know what's going on. If you need help, call them; they are very good resources. I consider myself lucky that I am allowed to do this work I love without being a veterinarian or having a college degree, and I am very grateful every day that these agencies allow me to work hands-on with wildlife.

The rules are in place for a reason. One example in our State is the "10-mile" rule, meaning an animal must be released within 10 miles of the place it was found. This can be tricky sometimes, especially if an animal comes to you without paperwork or if the area is under development, or is otherwise not a good release site. If the 10-mile rule can't be done, we are allowed to obtain permission from the State to find another suitable release site.

The 10-mile rule is in place for several reasons. One reason is that the animal might have a mate, breeding site, and/or an established hunting area; basically territoriality, in a given area. Some birds and animals breed for life so we make our best efforts to keep mates together if we can. We don't want to introduce an animal into another animal's territory and have an animal chased out. We'd rather take that animal back home, where it already has an established territory.

This rule is also in place to help prevent the spread of disease. We don't want to release a sick animal into a healthy area and we don't want to release a healthy animal into a sick area. We definitely don't want to spread disease around the State, diseases like chronic wasting disease, etc.

Don't hoard animals. If you're not licensed for them, send them to someone who is. If you want to care for that kind of animal, get a license for it.

There are rules regarding particular animal rehab and release. We might not always like them, agree with them, or understand them but they're probably in place for a good reason.

WORKING WITH OTHER REHABILITATORS

It might take you years to find another rehabber or few that you can work well with. Rehabbers can help you. Rehabbers can drive you nuts! Personalities, philosophies, and work styles differ from person to person. A good and helpful rehabber is a rare find and can be worth their weight in gold. Some rehabbers can be very helpful because they care most about helping you help animals and they want you to be the best you can be, for the sake of the animals. Rehabbers can be very critical and judgmental, sometimes forgetting what it was like when they were new and starting out. Rehabbers can become cranky and burnt out, like me. Rehabbers can become your lifesavers. I myself believe that we are all learning something new every single day and there are really very few "experts" in this kind of work. I believe we should share what we know if it will help other rehabbers help the animals. And I believe that when a person thinks they know everything, they have ceased to learn anything.

People get into wildlife rehab for a variety of reasons, it seems. Most really, really want to help wildlife. Some really, really want to help people that find wildlife as well as helping animals. Some people are upwardly mobile in the animal care field and obtain their permits because it looks good on a resume. Some people have the misguided belief that this is glamorous work (again, volunteering at a wildlife rehab facility and cleaning up poop all day can certainly bring you promptly back to reality!)

I feel it is important to maintain professionalism when working with ALL people, including other rehabbers. During certain times of the year, usually in the fall when rehabbers are broke and exhausted and are preparing to begin year-end paperwork, we are usually short-tempered and don't even want to deal with another person or phone call, and it can be very difficult to be polite. There will always be gossip and back-biting, but we need to stick with our mission statements and think about why we're doing what we're doing; trying to help the animals.

Rehabilitators might sometimes need to watch each other's animals or trade animals, depending on facilities and resources. It isn't at all unusual for animals to go from one rehabber to another but we are very careful with regard to transfer of animals between facilities and in the case of some mammals, we keep our wildlife officers informed of transfers between facilities.

We try to help each other out when we can. However, we must be very respectful of the other rehabbers' time and resources. If we get a donation with an animal that we end up taking to another rehabber, we should send that donation with that animal. If we can, and sometimes we simply can't, but if we can we should try to send food and supplies with that animal to go to that other rehabber, too. Available resources should stay with the animal.

If we need help from another rehabber we should call around until we find the help we need. Some will help us, some won't. We don't ask another rehabber to break the law for us. I try to help other rehabbers if they need it but I will not break the laws to help them or give them advice on how to care for an animal they shouldn't have in the first place.

If we need another rehabber to take our animal, it is up to us to make the transport arrangements; not the accepting rehabber's job. If we aren't able to do this, then maybe the accepting rehabber can help us with that. Other rehabbers are just as busy as we are, maybe even busier, and they are doing us a huge favor by taking over the care of our animal. We need to be respectful of their time and situation. We need to make the transition as easy as possible on everyone involved.

Sending rehabber also needs to send written information, in particular the animal intake form, to the accepting rehabber that came with the animal and it is our job to make every effort we can to ensure that we DO get paperwork with that animal, so the animal can be released where it was found and so that the accepting rehabber can obtain more information if needed from the people that found the animal originally.

As the accepting rehabber it is our job to not take animals we can't take care of. Some rehabbers just can't say NO when they are full, and this doesn't help the animals or anyone else. As the accepting rehabber I feel it is my job to keep the sending rehabber posted as to the status of their animal during its stay at my facility, if they're interested.

I also feel I must address the issue of ticking someone off. It's not a matter of if; it's definitely a matter of when. After conducting my own informal survey, I have found that many of us have the gift of putting our foot in our mouth, or saying something to another rehabber that we don't really mean or is taken out of context. We realize this months down the road when the other rehabber won't call us back or there's some other form of miscommunication. We just know we're never going to figure out what it is we said or did. So please, please, please if we tick you off let us know so we can fix it! Rehabbers are usually doing a million things at once, including talking, and it's very easy to say the wrong thing if we're distracted and not really thinking about what we're saying. If you don't want to deal with us by phone or in person, e-mail us! We don't go out of our way to offend but for some of us, it's just a gift. And I personally don't have an attention span long enough that allows me to carry a grudge.

Overall I feel that in order to benefit the animals and the people that care for them, we need to communicate as best as we can and try to get along as best as we can. Even if we have personality conflicts and just simply don't get along, we have to put all of that aside for the best interest of the animals. There have been times when other rehabbers that I know can't stand me have sent me animals to care for because they knew it was the right thing to do for the animals' sake. I have a fresh appreciation for them and a new respect; they put their personal feelings aside in the best interest of that animal. If we can't deal with each other on the phone or in person, there's always good ol' e-mail!

VALUE THE
VETERINARIANS AND STAFF

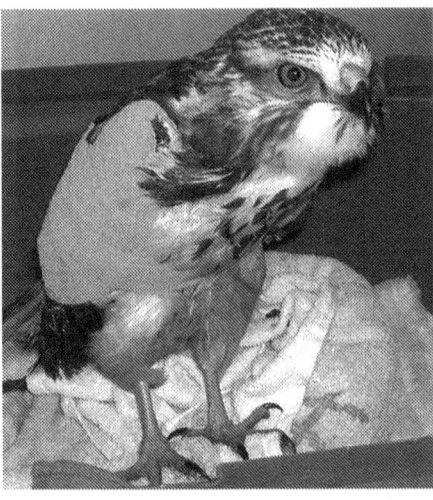

Young Swainson's hawk.

It has been my experience that the veterinarians and staff almost always donate their time and services. Some might charge a small fee for medicine or diagnostics, but overall these caregivers are tremendously helpful and valuable, and we mustn't abuse them.

Veterinarians are like everybody else; some you'll work well with and others you might not work so well with. You need to find a good veterinarian that you can work well with and communicate well with.

Veterinarians and veterinary staff that donate their time and services caring for wildlife aren't getting paid for this. Their paying customers must ALWAYS come first. We shouldn't barge in whenever we feel like it, demanding service and acting like we're the experts-because we're not. We may have a little more knowledge in some areas than the vet but we must respect their time, their training, and their willingness to help. If they need our help, they'll ask for it. We should wait our turn patiently. We can listen and ask questions instead of talking. If we abuse our veterinarians, we might find they no longer wish to help us.

We can help by not bringing every single animal to the vet. This is really difficult when we're new and starting out because we aren't always sure what condition necessitates a trip to the vet. With time and experience we become better able to assess who needs to see the doctor and who doesn't. The vets can help us with this. And we can help the vet by letting them know what animals we're licensed for and can accept. We can help the vet by keeping our animals contained and doing the handling of the animal, if the vet isn't comfortable or able to do so. We can help the vet by picking up an animal when we say we are going to and not let it languish at the vet clinic. Veterinary hospitals are very busy places and they probably don't have the time to feed baby birds or critical wild animals, and it's not their fault if the animal dies because it wasn't picked up when it was supposed to be. They're employees, on the clock, and must take care of their paying patients.

If we ask an animal finder to bring their animal to the vet, then it is our job to follow through and if that animal needs a pick-up, it is our job to arrange that pick-up. We don't dump animals at the vet and then wash our hands of the situation. If an animal finder is particularly difficult to deal with and will create a problem for the vet (as in they expect veterinary care but think the wild animal will be going home with them) then it is our job to inform that person of how it works and that the animal will NOT be going home with them from the vet. If necessary we might need to get the critter picked up ourselves and take that animal to the vet. We're not law enforcement and if an animal finder doesn't want to relinquish that animal, I give their phone number to my wildlife officer, who IS law enforcement, and let him or her handle the situation. We don't place ourselves, volunteers, provisionals, veterinarians and staff, or anyone else in harm's way if we can avoid it.

We can help the veterinarian by making sure they have intake forms available to be completed upon intake of the animals. You're going to need this paperwork for a variety of reasons, including year-end reporting for license renewal as well as release information for your animal. The paperwork is so very important.

We can help the veterinarian by providing our own transport containers for the animals we pick up. This is good for us also because it means our kennel will be going home with us!

Keep in mind that not all veterinarians treat all kinds of birds and animals. Before we show up at a vet clinic with an animal we should call ahead if we can and see if they're available to help us. We need to know what animals they will help us with.

We are very fortunate to work with a wonderful avian veterinarian in town; the guy that taught us the "less is more" style of wildlife care that has worked very well for our patients. But he doesn't treat bats, porcupines, and other mammals. We work with a few wonderful reptile vets in town and a gifted mammal vet in the Englewood area. And we have excellent quality of care from the emergency animal clinics in town, with very caring staff and the willingness to learn new things, and one of whom is the only vet I've ever worked with that addresses pain management in wildlife. Sometimes you might be REALLY lucky and find a vet that will make house calls.

We can help ourselves, the wildlife, the veterinarians, and the staff by being respectful of their time. We can help the veterinarians and staff by being courteous and maintaining professionalism. We can help the veterinarians and staff by being respectful and polite, valuing their experience and knowledge. We can help the veterinarians and staff, and everyone who helps us, by saying Thank You, either verbally, with a nice card, food, etc.

I think we find that if we are considerate of the people that help us, we're more likely to get the help we need when we need it, and sometimes even more help than we ever expected.

WORKING WITH THE PUBLIC

My own personal belief is that wildlife rehab is just as much about helping people as it is about helping the wildlife they find. You'll appreciate this better when a hysterical woman brings you a convulsing poisoned pigeon or a distraught commuter shows up with a bloody car-hit fox or worse yet, with an animal they accidentally injured themselves or their pet did. Both the animal finder and the animal need your help. Don't be rude.

We rehabbers are quick to call ourselves "animal people" and usually we prefer working with animals over working with people. But like it or not, working with people is something that is part of this job. We can't do wildlife rehab without working with people. And whether we're on the private list or the public list, people are going to find us, and we need to be polite and helpful, and that can be a real challenge at times!

People will call us if they need help with an animal. People will call us because they're bored and want to talk about the weather. People will call to see if we have a Chihuahua for sale. People will call us because they don't want their guinea pig anymore and want us to take it. They'll call us because there's a dead bird on their lawn and they want us to come get it. People will call us for many, many different reasons. I work full-time and can't be on the phone all day or I'd get fired from my job and have to live in my car! I don't answer my phone but check the messages very, very frequently. I prioritize the phone calls and return them immediately if it's regarding an urgent wildlife situation. The others have to wait until after work and the Chihuahua people will wait until my day off, during busy season.

Essentially people call us because they need help. I help people with their pet issues by referring them to low-cost spay and neuter facilities, and help them find low-cost medical care for their animal, if such is available. I spend a large part of my time talking people OUT of getting a pet when it appears they aren't physically, financially, or otherwise able to make that commitment. I refer people that are able to make the lifetime commitment to an animal to adopt from legitimate animal shelters.

Pets aren't my business and I know I don't have to help people with pet problems. But you know what? I feel that helping people IS my business, and so I make it a personal practice to return every phone call (if they leave me a phone number and most of it's not missing, which usually happens when they call on a cell phone!) Each call has value and needs to be handled in a timely manner if possible; again, that can be a real challenge during busy baby season. I let people know I'm much quicker to reach by e-mail than phone most times. My dream is of having volunteer help to retrieve the messages and put out the fires while I am at work!

Does the critter even need to come to rehab in the first place? A little bit of time spent on the phone determining if the animal really needs rescue can prevent a lot of time and resources being used for animal that comes to rehab that doesn't need to. During baby season I find it entirely worthwhile to spend 30 minutes or so on the phone with someone who has found a baby because if we can reunite the baby with its mother, preventing the need to come to rehab in the first place, then everyone benefits; the animal, me, and the finder of the animal, who feels they have accomplished a wonderful thing.

We do need to think about liability and not ask the public to do anything risky or dangerous. We don't want them getting injured. If they've already picked up the bat and played with it for a week before calling us, then we need to let them know it's up to them to call their physician and the Health Department right away.

I feel it is my duty to educate callers about the risks of handling wildlife and I feel it is my duty to inform them of the laws regarding possession of wildlife; how else would they know? I find the vast overwhelming majority of people don't know it's against the law to possess wildlife, let alone the feather they find blowing around their yard. They need to know that birds and mammals can carry parasites, worms, and disease. They need to know that some animals can carry rabies. They need to know that they, their family, and their pets can be injured by wildlife. And that brings me to another topic that is still SO hard to deal with-people that don't want to give up their critter.

In our State possession of wildlife is illegal without proper permits. People call here because they want to know how to care for a wild animal they want to keep. Usually they've had it a while and it's not doing well. I inform them, gently, of the fact the animal needs help, they're not legally allowed to have it, and that no veterinarian is going to help them because they're not a legal possessor of that animal, and how getting that animal to a licensed rehabber is the best thing for that animal to get the help it needs. Most times they see the light and will turn their animal over to rehab. But sometimes they absolutely, positively will not because they're attached. At that point my only recourse is to let them know I'm giving their contact information to my wildlife officer and he or she will be paying them a visit to confiscate that animal. This isn't how I like to handle it but what else can I responsibly do?

We see again and again and again that someone found an animal, think they know how to care for it, and then it begins to fail. Now they're looking for help. They don't understand why bird seed isn't good for an owl, why fast food isn't good for baby foxes, or why milk and oatmeal aren't good for baby birds. They just can't believe that tiny ducklings shouldn't be placed in the swimming pool; after all, they're water birds, right? They don't understand the tragic consequences of making a fawn into a neighborhood pet. Instead of getting really angry and reading them the riot act, we try to squelch our feelings of frustration and view this as an opportunity to provide some education and help this person to understand. I know that if a person has a bad experience with a rehabber they are not going to look for help the next time they find an animal. I'm amazed at the number of "repeat" business we get. My hope is that they'll gain something positive from the experience of working with us, even if the outcome isn't what they expected and they don't get the results they were seeking, and that they will remember us and call us if they need help again. I treat each and every contact with a member of the community as a potential opportunity for outreach and education.

Treat the Public courteously and with respect. After all, if wasn't for the Public bringing us animals, we wouldn't be able to do this work we love.

OH, NO; I'M FALLING APART!

Please take good care of you! This kind of work takes a toll on our bodies. We work very hard and are exposed to disease, injury, stress, and the day-to-day physical labor. Many rehabbers drop out the first year, due to a variety of reasons, with physical ailments and stress being a couple of them.

Stress is a fact of life. Some of us deal with it by eating, some by shopping (like we can afford to!) and some by dropping out. Again this is why I feel it is so important to know your limitations. If you can care for only 2 animals a year and do a good job, and feel good about it and stay healthy, providing those 2 animals excellent care, then yay for you. I think about how the animals and we rehabbers would benefit if there were lots of rehabbers, each caring for just a few each year instead of a few rehabbers caring for a few hundred each year. Don't let the guilt get to you. Other rehabbers can guilt-trip you into saying Yes when you really need to say No. If you destroy yourself, you are no good to you, the animal, or anyone else. In this line of work there really are no days off and nobody but another rehabber truly understands what we deal with. Hopefully we have someone-another rehabber is good—that we can vent on, someone that knows it's just exhaustion and stress speaking, and doesn't take it personally.

Sheer exhaustion is another reality of wildlife rehab. Some rehabbers are up around the clock feeding babies or caring for critical critters, and/or are doing this around their full-time regular paying job and family duties. The summer can blow by in a fog, while we work in zombie mode. I think of a wonderful rehabber that works her regular full-time job in addition to doing an amazing job with several hundred baby birds and animals each year. I think of the rehabber who is my former sponsor, a lady who is up round-the-clock with baby mammals, working, raising her kids, pet-sitting, and caring for an elderly woman each week that's a considerable distance away as well as providing excellent care to the wildlife in her care. These women take the time to help the rest of us with our questions and situations. I honestly and truly don't know how these ladies do it, but they're my heroes! The rest of us give lousy job performance at work and count the days until November, looking for a day we can just sleep the whole day, or even sleep in until daylight! I thank God every day for my amazing, understanding, and very patient boss.

Illness is a reality we must deal with. I think we all know that keeping birds in the house is very hazardous to our health. This can cause serious respiratory problems and is the reason some rehabbers must drop out. We need to be aware of fleas and ticks, and worms as well; in particular, the raccoon roundworm. We're exposed to any number of zoonotic diseases and other agents. We must always be so very careful to take care of ourselves and quarantine the best we can. We should have a good communication with our primary care physician and inform them of the work we do, so if we get sick they are better able to help us. I personally keep updated on my tetanus vaccine and am preparing to have the rabies series very soon. I keep the animals out of my house if I can. I take vitamins and my prescription medications.

Don't feel bad about saying NO if you need to. And don't feel guilty about taking some time off if you need to. If you're lucky enough to get a vacation, hooray for you! I know you definitely need one. If you need to take a year or two off to tend to yourself and your family, you'll either come back to rehab refreshed and revitalized or you will have decided this work is simply not worth what it does to your quality of life. You may realize that continuing wildlife rehab will do permanent damage to your health and your personal relationships. Overall, you must take care of YOU and please do!

LIABILITY

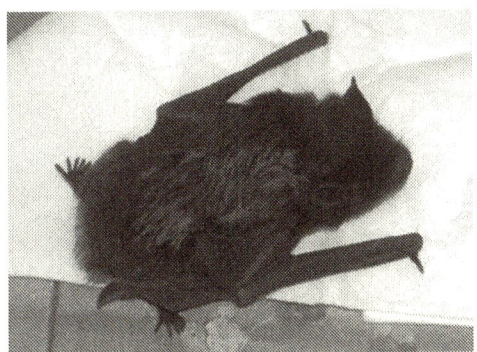

Silver-haired bat

I'm just going to touch very lightly on this subject, as it is very complex and detailed. You will definitely need to do some research on liability as a home-based wildlife rehabber. Before committing to rehab, you might want to call your homeowner's insurance company and find out if they will still insure you if you keep animals in your home. I found out the hard way that my insurance company drops people that keep birds, ferrets, and/or reptiles in their homes. You need to be very honest and up-front with your insurance company because if you lie to them and have an incident, you will probably be out of luck. Find an insurance company that is on-board with what you do. It will cost you more; mine is double now.

You need insurance to protect yourself, your home and assets, and people. What if someone gets bitten or injured from an animal in your rehab care? What if a volunteer or someone you're sponsoring becomes sick or injured from working with wildlife? Keep these possibilities in mind when you're having such a hard time finding someone to sponsor YOU, and be prepared to sign a waiver of liability as a provisional. What if you tell a homeowner to pick up the raccoon and put it in a box, and they get bitten? What if you tell someone to pick up a bat and bring it to your house, and find out later the bat has rabies?

This is very scary stuff and nobody ever, ever talked about it when I was new and starting out. This is a very important consideration and I absolutely feel it must be addressed. The consequences if you're not prepared can potentially be devastating.

This takes us back to why wildlife rehab isn't necessarily a "sharing" experience for you to allow your friends and family members to play with your animals, or cart the poor animals to the schools or other places. If your animals need care and you're on a schedule, find a legal critter-sitter or stay home. Take sick or injured animals directly to the vet or your facility, and hit the errands later on. Don't be dragging them all over the place for show-and-tell. This is illegal, detrimental to the animal, and if something bad happens, guess who could potentially be liable? Yep, that would be YOU!

I recommend investigating additional insurance coverage if you can afford it. If you can't afford it, be very, very careful.

BIRDS, AND MAMMALS, AND REPTILES; OH MY!

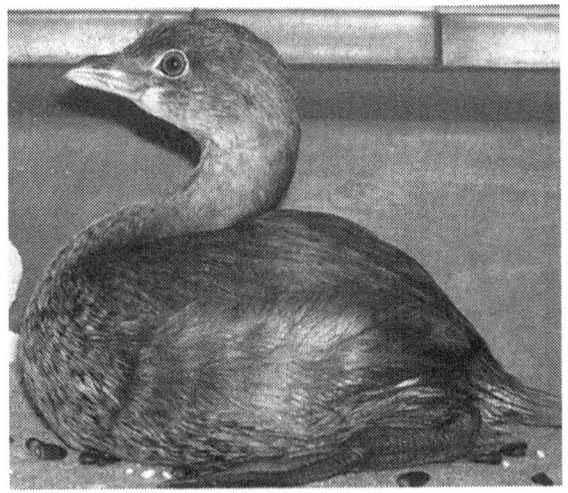

Pied-billed grebe

So just what is your passion? Blue jays? Bears? Mountain lions? Owls? Snakes and turtles? Bats? Deer and elk? Some people rehab a large variety of animals. Some take only squirrels, or bats, or turtles, or whatever they're most comfortable with. With time you'll find your specialty or niche. I always thought I'd live life and die as the cat lady. I was told yesterday morning by a woman that showed up on my porch with an injured sparrow that I'm considered "the bird lady of Ellicott;" who'd have thunk? Truth be told, I consider myself a rabbit and owl person.

The beauty of wildlife rehab in Colorado is it's up to you and your resources. You won't be caring for mountain lions in your Denver condo or bears in your Pueblo duplex. You won't (and shouldn't) be raising squirrels in your college dorm.

Licensing can be difficult to obtain in residential areas because of zoning. Also there is the consideration of the care and housing guidelines we are required to follow. Maybe you can't build an outdoor cage in your back yard because the city won't allow it but perhaps you have a basement or a spare bedroom in the back of the house that you can set up as an infirmary for critical patients or babies that would go on to other rehab facilities later, when they're ready for the larger facilities. This is again where knowing zoning rules in your area and your limitations is important. If you're limited to caring for just a few babies to send to another rehabber later on to finish the process, that's fantastic. People like me can't take babies because of my work schedule so people that can take babies and send to me when they're self-feeding is a good thing. If you need larger facilities than you are able to provide at your home and/if you can't build outdoor enclosures for the animals in your care, you might want to find another rehabilitator that will give you access to their outdoor enclosures for prerelease training when they're ready. You might need to provide this other rehabber's name on your rehab application.

We are inspected by the State DOW and need to pass inspection before obtaining our permits. In Colorado a State permit from the Colorado Division of Wildlife is required for all bird and mammal rehabilitation permits, and a Federal rehab permit is required for all migratory birds. Your sponsor will likely help you with all the nuts and bolts of this but overall, be realistic in what you think zoning and your resources will allow.

You might hear the term "glamour species" bandied about. I've been doing this a long time and still don't understand the term. To me, poop is poop, with none of it being more glamorous than the other. I can't imagine cleaning up moose poop is any more glamorous than cleaning up raccoon poop. I know cleaning up owl poop isn't any more glamorous than cleaning up pigeon poop.

Now, about those nuts and bolts..... .

STARTING OUT

I wholeheartedly recommend you do some volunteering before pursuing your rehab permit. Probably nobody will sponsor you if you don't and there's a really good reason for that-volunteering can be a good test to determine your level of commitment.

For some reason, people think we sit around and play with animals all day. They want to sign their 4-year-old up for volunteer service. Translated, that means that they want their 4-year-old to play with the wildlife. We don't allow that at our facility. They want their friends, family, co-workers, pool dude, and the landscape guys to share in the joy of wildlife rehab, as if this is glamorous work and the animals enjoy being manhandled and eyeballed to death. I am here to tell you this is definitely not glamorous work. This is drudgery. And I have to say it for the millionth time, not something for small children to participate in on a hands-on level! Animals aren't toys. And we don't want the kids getting sick or injured. I don't believe you can have a full appreciation of what wildlife rehab is until you've done some volunteering.

Your volunteer work won't consist of walking lions on a leash in your stilettos or frolicking with bear cubs, just so you know. A potential responsible sponsor probably won't let you within 100 yards of their wildlife for quite some time. These animals don't know you and don't need to, right now. What a sponsor wants to determine is if you're dedicated to doing the dirty work. Will you clean poopy cages and kennels? Scrub dirty dishes? Hose off the dirty laundry? Help with the filing? Answer phones? Do some errands? If you want to slide right past the chores, don't expect to go into a flight cage and play with the eagle! You need to prove your commitment to the work before getting near the animals.

Once you've decided all the grunge work is something you can handle, and you've considered the prior information in this book, and once you've decided what types of critter you wish to provide care for, you might want to go to the Colorado Division of Wildlife web site or call their person in charge of special licensing to get some more information. She is a wonderful lady that will tell you what you need to know.

You will have plenty of material to review and get to know, you will need training, and the DOW is very good about answering your questions. Very simply put, you will need a Colorado licensed wildlife rehabilitator to sponsor you. You will need a minimum of one veterinarian that will provided donated services to you and says so in writing, as you are responsible for any and all costs incurred with wildlife rehabilitation. Ultimately you will have an inspection by the State of your facilities, to ensure you are equipped to responsibly care for the critters you're requesting permission to care for.

Currently, we are not required to have a college degree or be a veterinarian to be a licensed wildlife rehabilitator but there is plenty of education needed.

So are you scared yet?

YOUR NEW BEST FRIEND, YOUR SPONSOR

Once you have a Sponsor, you become a Provisional.

One of the first things you will need to do is find a licensed Colorado wildlife rehabilitator to sponsor you. Ideally you will want a sponsor in your area because this is the person you will be reporting each and every animal that comes into your hot little hands to. A sponsor is here to help you learn. A sponsor may require you to volunteer for them at first and this is entirely reasonable. As a sponsor we try to be flexible and considerate of your time and situation by not giving you a volunteer schedule you can't possibly keep. A good sponsor can be a challenge to find. Why, you ask? Remember that chapter on liability? We rehabbers live in fear that if we sponsor someone for rehab, they will become our worst nightmare and give us endless headaches. We need to be 1000% sure that you are not going to make our lives hell.

We rehabbers share stories and they will make your hair stand up! Provisionals that break the laws, provisionals that don't tell us what's going on, provisionals that try to make pets out of their wildlife, provisionals with rather bizarre ideals and philosophies, and on and on. You can understand why so many of us are hesitant to take on that responsibility. You will have to work very hard at showing a potential sponsor that you are not a loony tune and that you are truly dedicated to this work.

As a provisional you have very clear responsibilities to your sponsor. Some are the law, some are put in place by the sponsor themselves. If you don't follow the rules, you could be dropped like a hot potato and your animals taken away by wildlife officers. You need to notify your sponsor immediately when an animal comes to you. You need to keep detailed and meticulous paperwork on each and every single animal that comes to you for care, as you will need this for your licensing and so will your sponsor. You need to work very well with your sponsor and you need to communicate very well with your sponsor. You do not have Rehabilitator status on your permit until your sponsor releases you in writing to the State and to the Feds, at which time you will receive your Rehabilitator licenses. If you have any kind of problem with authority figures and/or someone telling you what to do, you may close this book and go watch TV. Wildlife rehab probably isn't for you.

YOU NEED A GOOD
VETERINARIAN OR FEW

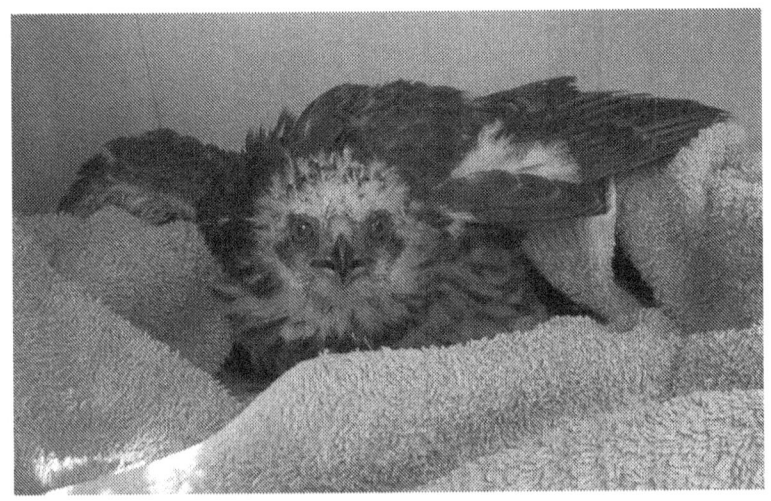

Young Cooper's Hawk

Maybe your sponsor can help you with this. Before you can apply for your permit you need to have a letter from the veterinarian or veterinarians that will treat wildlife for you.

You will want to find a veterinarian that is experienced in working with the animal you will be caring for. Ask around. Ask your sponsor, ask other rehabbers, and call some veterinarians; the closer to you, the better. Remember that not all veterinarians treat wildlife. They don't get paid to do it and they're busy with their paying clients.

Once you find some potential veterinarians, call and make an appointment to speak with them. Let them know who you are, who your sponsor is, and the type of help you need. Find out if they will donate their time and services, and if not, whether or not they offer a rehabber discount. Remember, YOU will be paying for all the expenses incurred in wildlife rehab, and medical care can be very, very expensive if not donated or discounted.

You will need a letter from the veterinarian to submit to the State with your application. Find out what you can do to make the process easier for the veterinarian. Don't drive the veterinarian nuts. And don't ask the veterinarian to treat your pets for free or a discount. Expect to pay full price, always, for services to your personal pets; dogs, cats, etc. Veterinarians communicate with each other just like rehabbers do, and if you become a problem, you'll have a hard time finding a veterinarian to help you.

Once you start getting animals, re-read the chapter on working with veterinarians!

INSPECTION TIME

Once you've done all that you need to do to get your wildlife rehab application together and once you have submitted your application, expect a visit from your potential wildlife officer.

They will interview you, and assess your knowledge and understanding in the areas of working with wildlife and wildlife rehab.

They will inspect your facilities in accordance with the species you have applied to care for. They want to be sure you can responsibly care for these animals. They want to see you're not going to keep animals in your living room or in a shoebox under your bed. They need to see and know that wild animals are not going to be exposed to the sights and sounds of you, your family, your pets, the TV, phone, radio, etc.

If you're fortunate enough to be able to keep animals outside, they will inspect to make sure your outdoor enclosures are the right size and configuration, according to predetermined requirements and standards. You won't be keeping vultures in a canary cage or bears in a chicken coop. The inspecting officer needs to see that your facilities are escape-proof and predator-proof. They need to see that they offer shade, shelter, sunlight, and protection. Your facilities must be well-lit and well-ventilated. You need to have proper food and supplies on-hand. You need to have a variety of facilities to accommodate the different species, sizes, ages, and disabilities you will be dealing with. Your cages need to be kept locked.

The inspection process is very important and is also a great opportunity to meet and get to know your wildlife officer. Now your officer submits their findings and recommendations to the Special Licensing Unit ...

SO WHERE'S MY PERMIT?

This is a government process. If the State approves your permit, you'll usually know very quickly. The current person in charge of Special Licensing at our Colorado Division of Wildlife is very thorough and very prompt. If your permit arrives, you can do the happy dance and take a deep breath. If your permit is denied, you'll need to find out why and what to do about it. Either way, inform your sponsor of your permit status immediately. The rehab community is very tight and probably your sponsor will be in touch with the DOW on a regular basis, and you absolutely want your sponsor to find out information from you, not from someone else.

If you have applied to care for migratory birds, once you have that State permit in your hands you must immediately apply to the US Fish and Wildlife Service for their rehabilitation permit as well. Your State permit means nothing without the accompanying Federal permit and vice versa. You need to get on that right away! Your Federal permit will take much longer to show up because the folks at USFWS are very overburdened, and up to their eyeballs in applications for several states and several different types of permits. Be patient; they're doing the best they can.

As a provisional you are working under your sponsor and answerable to your sponsor. A provisional cannot sponsor another rehabilitator.

A permit for raptors (birds of prey, not dinosaurs!) is a separate permit from your migratory bird permit, and a permit for eagles is yet another different permit. Your migratory bird permit does not allow you to rehabilitate these birds. You will need to complete a different application, undergo different training, build different facilities, and have a different inspection to rehabilitate hawks, owls, falcons, and yet another permit for the rehabilitation of eagles.

If you wish to rehab bats and/or spotted and hog-nosed skunks, you will have different State licensing requirements, including proof of current rabies titers. Your regular State mammal rehab permit does not allow you to rehab bats or skunks.

If you find yourself with an animal you're not licensed for, you need to IMMEDIATELY turn it over to someone who is. This is about the best interest of that animal, not about the fact that a golden eagle is a refreshing change from a robin or the spotted fawn is more interesting than the squirrels! If you get caught with animals you're not supposed to have, you risk losing your license and possibly fines. If you decide at some point you'd like to add another species to your rehab permit, you will go back through the application and inspection process. You need that permit BEFORE you take that animal. Don't ask another rehabber to help you care for an animal you're not supposed to have. And don't ever, ever underestimate the rehabber "grapevine."

"THE LIST"

Once you have your permit you will have the opportunity to decide if you want to be on a public list or only the private list of licensed wildlife rehabilitators.

The public list is exactly what the name implies; public. That means wildlife agencies have your name, number, and species licensed for and will call you if they need you. Your name and number will probably be floating around the Internet as well. Other rehabbers will have your name and number too, and will be calling you if (when) they need you. Basically, that public list is available to everyone. You will be amazed at how much your phone rings if you're on that public list. My sponsor was very wise and she advised me to not go on the public list the first year. She was absolutely right; I'd probably have been scared off and dropped out that first year! The private list is pretty much for the use of wildlife agencies.

Once you're on "the list" expect to be bombarded during baby season. Remember to know your limitations and say NO when you're up to your ears. Don't feel guilty; you're a name on a list and if you say no, the caller will move on to the next name on the list. You owe it to these animals to give them the best care you can and that means saying NO if you're maxed out.

In Colorado there is a very great need for rehabbers of baby birds and other small mammals. You can, if you allow it to happen, literally find yourself with 60 or more of these critters in your house in the space of a few days if you let it happen. Baby birds are the biggest challenge in my opinion because of the horrific feeding schedule-every 15 minutes, sunup to sundown. Baby squirrels and baby raccoons can be on a different feeding schedule; all day and overnight sometimes. If you are licensed to care for these animals, seriously consider BEFORE you're on the list how many you can handle. Don't collect 200 of them and then try to dump them on other rehabbers. It's not fair.

NOW I HAVE MY FIRST....

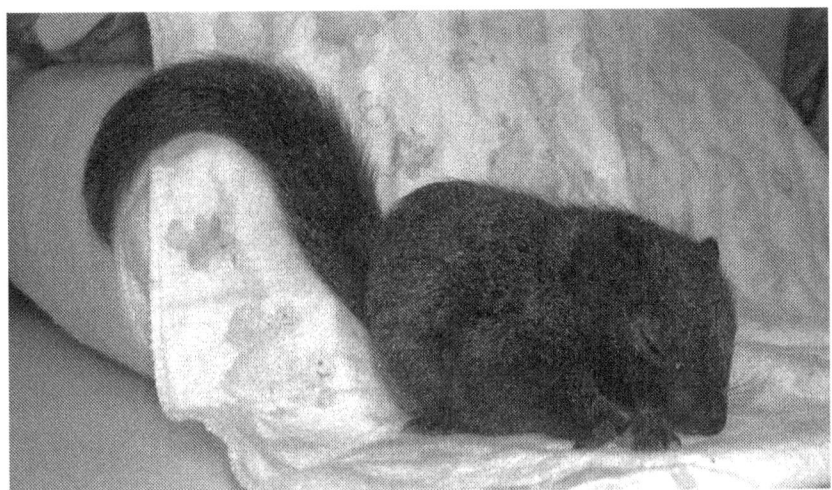

Young squirrel.

Okay, the veterinarian has called you to come and pick up the critter. Of course you will let the vet know when you will be there and you will be there when you're supposed to be there. You dig through your equipment to find the proper container for your animal and prepare the heat disc, if indicated. You rush over there to go pick up your patient. Get the intake information from the veterinarian before you leave so you don't forget. It might not be there later on. Listen to what the veterinarian tells you about the animal's condition and the treatment plan. Ask questions; don't be afraid. This is how you learn.

Now take that animal directly home. Don't stop on the way to get a pizza or run the kids around. Turn off the radio and don't smoke in the car. Go directly home-NOW! Once I get home, what I do next is place that animal WITHOUT HANDLING it in the dark, quiet room I have prepared and give it time to de-stress.

This is a good time to make a copy of your paperwork and send it to your sponsor right away. The sponsor might need that information to gather more information. Your sponsor must have that information for him or her on their permit to sponsor you. Now go and file your paperwork in a safe place where you can find it later on. You're going to need it to renew your license at the end of the year. Next you need to call your sponsor and let them know what you have, how it is, where it came from, what the vet said, etc. Ask questions. Don't be a wise-acre with your sponsor; we're here to help.

If the animal is brought to you directly from the finder you may or may not need to see the vet. I always called my sponsor first if I was unsure, and she was ultimately helpful in helping me determine if I needed to bother the vet with this animal. If I see exposed bone I go to the vet. If I see obvious horrible fractures or a missing eye, I go to the vet. If there's an obvious life-threatening injury like a fish hook embedded in the throat, I see the vet. If the animal sustained a car hit or fell out of the tree, I see the vet for a spinal/pelvic x-ray. No use keeping the animal suffering if it's back or neck is broken.

Ask your sponsor the questions you have. You might find yourself calling your sponsor a LOT with questions. Your sponsor expects this so don't worry about it. Sponsors worry most about the provisionals that DON'T ask questions and are very silent. Remember, you must communicate with your sponsor. Don't hide or disappear. If you're going to be unavailable for any reason you need to let your sponsor know. Now, about that animal.

... SO WHAT DO I DO NEXT?

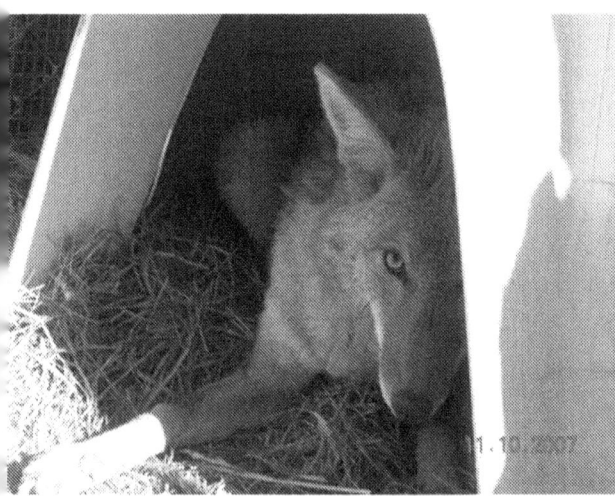

Car hit coyote

Now you have your first wild animal and I imagine you're SOOO excited; after all, who wouldn't be? Now the hard work begins.

Remember the part about putting the animal in the quiet, dark room to de-stress? That's what I do. I think they deserve it.

I don't yank it out of its container and play with it for hours. I don't drag it to the neighbor's house for show-and-tell or let the cat or dog sniff it. I don't let the kids manhandle it to death. Stress kills wildlife, and we'll address that later on.

Once some time has passed and the animal is calm, I go in and take a very quick picture. I use my pictures for a variety of reasons, not the least of which is identification purposes (I might need help identifying this bird) and also for a before-and-after, if the animal does well. I will take 1 or 2 pictures and I don't position the animal; it is kept where and how it is.

In the room alone, where it is quiet and peaceful, I can gently remove the animal from the container and do an exam. When you're new the exam might be fairly limited. Do you notice any strange smells or sounds? Is there fluid coming from the eyes/ears/mouth/orifices? Feel both arms/legs/wings simultaneously with your eyes closed or fixed on the ceiling. Are they symmetrical? Do you feel swelling/broken bones/crepitus?

This isn't a how-to-do-medical-care book so I will not go into detail about all the medical care details. For the exam and treatment of your animals, you will likely have plenty of help from your sponsor, other rehabbers, and the veterinarians. And keep your mind open. My hope is that you will see each animal as an individual and that you will learn with each one.

Make sure the animal is comfortable. Provide heat if needed. Provide fluids safely if needed. Ask for help if you need it. Now leave that critter be for a while!

IS IT SOMETHING I DID?

I'll address this right now, rather than later. Your animal might be dead when you go to check on it the first/second/third time. You might get up bright and early in the morning to go tend to your patient and find it has passed.

The sad reality is that animals die. They can die overnight. They can die on your front porch as you reach for their container. They can die while they're eating. They can die when they look really good. They can even drop dead in your hands. And you will always wonder if it's something you did or didn't do. Learn from each one and try to not repeat mistakes.

Most likely it isn't something you did. Remember what these animals went through before someone picked them up; before someone found help, before someone brought that animal to you or the vet; the stress, fear, starvation and pain.

Now think about what the animal went through after it was found; the fear of being eaten by predators (that would be us, our kids, our pets,) the ride in the car, the experience of being in a vet clinic surrounded by lights, noise, and other animals; the stress of handling and the exam, and the treatment, then back in the car, and back to our home. I like to give animals a very peaceful reception when I get them here; I give them peace and quiet. They need it.

Sometimes the animal has internal damage that couldn't have been spotted, let alone fixed. An animal full of puncture wounds from cat teeth and claws, with broken air sacs, doesn't tend to do very well. You can't do anything about those air sacs surgically or chemically. And in cat attacks, you will probably never see blood.

So after all of this, we can appreciate what a truly special celebration a release is! Several days/weeks/months later when you take your photo of a happy, healthy animal on release days you can appreciate the miracle.

But what if you did everything exactly as you were supposed to and the animal died? Sit down and think about it. Wipe your tears, have some good chocolate and/or ice cream, and really think about what you could have done differently. Maybe it would have made a difference, maybe not. But learn everything you can from the experience and remember, sometimes the best thing we can offer an injured animal in pain is a peaceful passing. At least it was safe from predators and the elements, and it was comfortable.

And no, you may not keep the body-that's another permit! Ask your sponsor what to do with the body.

MY THOUGHTS ON EUTHANASIA

If death is too hard for you, this might not be the kind of work for you. We see lots of horrible things and it doesn't get much easier. Some of us develop a twisted and morbid sense of humor to deal with it. Some drop out because they just simply can't deal with it. I believe that death is the only sure thing in life and it has to be dealt with. Remember for every one that died there are several that still need you and still have a chance. You need to keep it together for those that have an opportunity to succeed.

If an animal has been abused and we are able to provide information on the abuser, we report it. If a bird has been shot, poisoned, or electrocuted, we report it.

With time, lots and lots of time, we become better able to determine what animal is a candidate for euthanasia. We look for signs of improvement. We look for quality of life. The decision for euthanasia can be difficult if the animal has some good days and some bad days; the good days give you so much hope and the bad days make you want to jump in the car and head to the vet for euthanasia (for the animal, not you!)

I feel that sometimes the very best gift we can make to an animal in pain and suffering is the gift of euthanasia. As hard as it is for us, it's pretty hard on the person that found that animal originally. I make absolutely no promises to people about the animal's potential for release. How in the world would I be able to know? If people want to know, tell them. If they don't want to know, don't tell them. Animal finders will wonder if it's something THEY did, and they will wonder if bringing the animal for help was even the right thing to do. These telephone calls are the worst calls to make but this is also an opportunity to let the animal finder know why bringing the animal for help is the right thing, even if the outcome isn't what they had hoped for.

I feel there is good euthanasia and bad euthanasia. This is just something I can see and feel. Euthanasia, in my opinion, should be conducted in a quiet area at the vet, with chemical anesthesia first, and then the injection. I feel a good euthanasia is an instant death, not a long, drawn out, prolonged, horrible death. My avian vet in town is a master, as are the emergency vets in town, and some others. The animal is gone before the stethoscope can be placed to the chest. I think of the vet in town that cries with each and every death, and he's been a veterinarian for a long time. This man cares so much about these animals. I figure if it's that hard for him, and he sees so much more of it than I do, then it's okay for me to have a breakdown, too. Be prepared for the fact that euthanasia in reptiles can take longer than in birds and mammals, due to slow metabolism.

You might have to shop around for euthanasia. And I won't address at-home euthanasia. There are things we are allowed to do at home and things we are not allowed to do at home. The things I'm allowed to do at home aren't things I'm comfortable with yet and the at-home methods of euthanasia in my opinion are pretty gruesome and not particularly efficient or humane, so my euthanasias happen at the vet. Talk to other rehabbers and the DOW about at-home death management if you're not located near a vet or if you want to do it at home. **We are not allowed to have the euthanasia drug.**

STRESS KILLS!

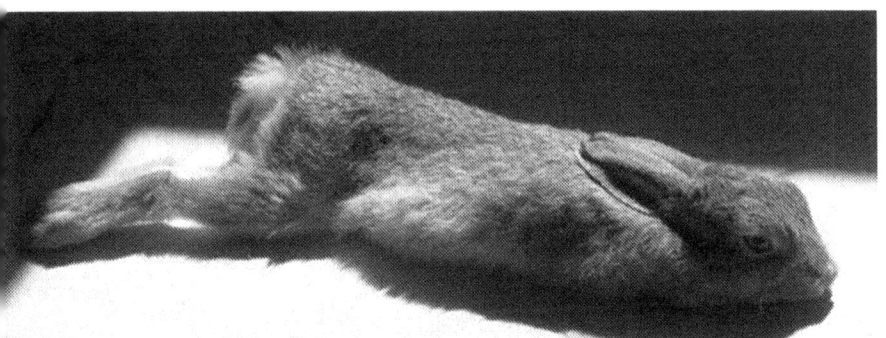

Cottontails can be very easily stressed.

We might think of stress as related to our jobs, family situations, social lives, health and money problems, and so forth. For wildlife in our care, stress is their lives, I believe.

My priority upon receiving wildlife is the de-stress. I feel the animal must feel calm and semi-safe before I can even hope to do a successful exam or treatment.

Animals are stressed by strange situations, sounds, sights, smells. Leave the perfume off, the air freshener off, and all that smelly stuff far, far away when dealing with animals. Don't smoke around your animals. When doing cleaning, place the animal outside in its container, in a secure place, so you can use your bleach and other cleaning products. Birds are very efficient breathers due to air sacs and sucking up chemical fumes can kill them.

Animals are stressed by pain. I still wonder, after all these years, why pain management is such a non-addressed element of what we do. When I used to ask many years ago, I got the standard reply: "A pain-free animal will just make its injuries worse." That could be true, but I haven't experienced that. I feel that some animals might give up on life because they can't deal with the pain. Once I finally found a decent pain management for rabbits, my rabbits started doing better. Same for other animals. I am very grateful for the veterinarian that responsibly administers the pain management before sending the animal home with me.

Animals are stressed by handling of humans. You're going to hear this again and again because I see it in my work over and over. I'm guessing animals view us as very big predators, what with our big round eyes in front of our heads and the sheer size, noise, and smell of us! That poor critter is probably thinking you're going to eat him. The animal is sitting quietly in your hand not because he loves you, as so many people seem to think, but because he is paralyzed by fear. I figure he might be thinking that if he makes himself real small and still, maybe I'll go away. Again I emphasize this isn't an opportunity to introduce the critter to your dog/cat/ferret. This isn't a squeeze-fest for your 3-year-old, either. I mention these things only because I've SEEN them, on more than one occasion. Excessive handling causes stress, can ruin feathers and fur. If you need to play with animals, go get a (legal) pet.

KIDS AND WORKING WITH WILDLIFE

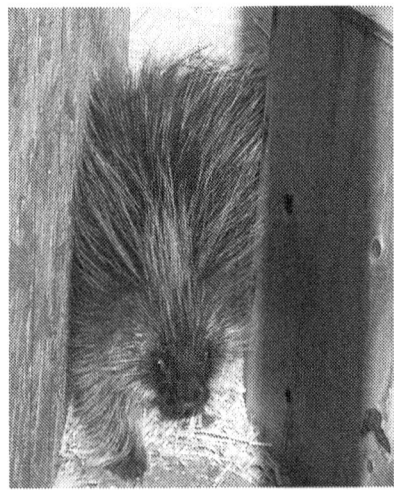

Porcupine

By now you must be thinking I don't allow kids near my wildlife in rehab. And you are absolutely, totally correct. That would be illegal and also not good for the animals. I work with children in my volunteer programs and I work with children in educational programs with raptors but children are never, ever allowed to get close enough to my animals to get harmed or to do harm. Kids are allowed to see my program birds from a safe distance. My program birds were born and raised in the wild, not raised from babies and tamed or otherwise imprinted. They are still wild and unlicensed people are not allowed to touch them. My animals in rehab are not on display.

Kids LOVE animals, and that's a fact of life. I feel that parents and adults need to teach children very early on about animals and life and responsibility. I feel that kids need to learn that animals are living creatures, not toys, and if we choose to live with them then we need to value their lives and take very, very good care of them. Animals don't have a choice or a voice; we do, and they depend on us.

Easter is my worst time of year. Impulse animal purchases aren't usually a good thing for the animals. I wish live animals were hidden in retailer basements at Easter, not heaped in front of the cash registers like the living sacrifices they are. If any thought was ever put into adopting an animal and if the majority of pet owners were responsible, there wouldn't be so many animals filling up the shelters and being euthanized.

It drives me nuts when I get the phone calls where someone wants me to take their bunnies/puppies/kittens because now they have too many and want to get rid of them. When I ask why the original animal wasn't neutered in the first place, I get the answer "I wanted my child to experience the wonder of life." I assume they mean the experience of watching an animal give birth. Rent a video. What about the rest of the life process? Now that the child has experienced reproduction, how about finishing the process of life and reproduction by showing these children what happens to these animals AFTER that "miracle of life?" I live for the day when people teach their children about responsible animal care, about the benefit to all animals when pets are neutered and not reproducing all over the place, and about the wonderful gift an animal contributes to our quality of life; how they deserve respect. I look forward to the day when the shelters are almost empty because people are doing the right thing. What would a child think about all those animals in cages at the local shelter? What would a parent tell that child when asked where did all these animals come from, and why are they here, and what is going to happen to them? How about let's teach children to value and appreciate ALL life?

Okay, now, about wildlife and working with children. Children love animals, there's no doubt about that. We do wish to share with them our wildlife, one of our most precious natural resources. So how can we do that responsibly, when there are animals living in our homes, as home-based rehabbers? Since I don't have children and am not experienced in doing rehab from home with kids in the house, I recommend talking with other rehabbers that do have kids in the home and find out how they do it.

Think about your child's safety first. At first you might not know what's wrong with that animal. It might be sick. It might have chemical poisoning. What are you exposing your child (and others) to? What about parasites; fleas, ticks, and worms? What if your mammal, unbeknownst to you, turns out to have rabies and has sneezed in your child's face? Your child might require serious medical care after an exposure. What if that wild animal bites, scratches, grabs your child with its talons or stabs your child with its long, pointed beak? What if an animal slaps your child with its quilled tail? (No, for the hundredth time, they CANNOT THROW QUILLS!) But they do shed them like hair.

Think about what you might bring home to your own pet. This is why your facilities are inspected so thoroughly. And there are reasons why children aren't allowed to become wildlife rehabbers.

I think that sharing wildlife work with children can be a beautiful thing when done responsibly. We know that children are visual and want to see animals. I find that once a child has the opportunity to see an animal, like the pets at home, they tend to lose interest pretty quickly.

I don't have children so I don't know what it's like to do wildlife rehab from home when there are kids in the house. I imagine the kids are very interested in what came from the vet and do want to see. Maybe their curiosity could be sated by a picture of the animal along with an explanation of what happened to it, the prognosis, and why the animal is in that quiet room with the door closed and locked along with the reasons why we need to respect the animals' need for peace and quiet? Maybe once the animal is moved outside the children might get a quick peek from a safe distance.

I once saw a facility where there was a 2-way glass window on the rehab room. This allows the animals the privacy they need while the rehabber could check in on them in a stress-free way. Maybe that would be an option for a home-based rehabber with kids in the house? It's something to consider.

KEEPING YOUR CRITTER COMFORTABLE

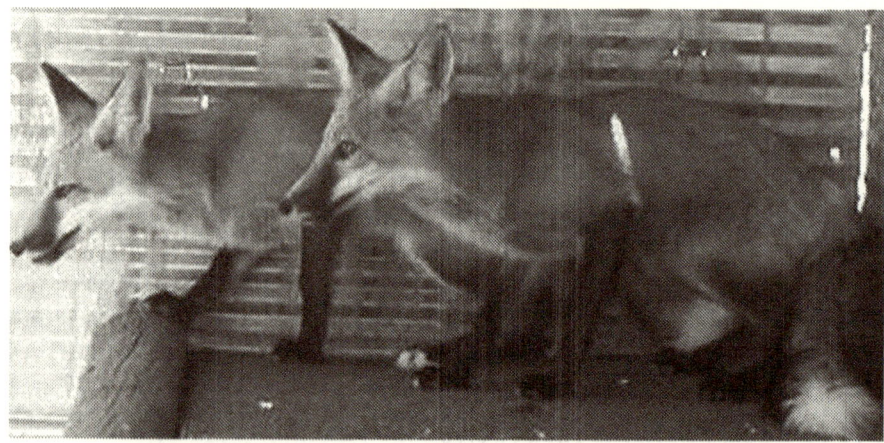

Foxes

At different times animals seem to need different things. This varies on their condition upon arrival at your facility. Some will be in very bad shape and will benefit from a dark and quiet situation. Some will be feeling quite chipper and may need a little stimulation by being near the window, to look out and see the sights. Some do better with others of their own kind nearby; not necessarily in the container with them. Some just need quality time in an outdoor enclosure, enjoying the sunshine, rain, moon and stars, and the fresh air. This is assessed at my facility on a case-by-case basis. Your sponsor can be very helpful in helping you determine the best situation for your critter.

This is also why the officer inspecting your facilities will need to see what you can provide animals of varying species, and their sizes, ages, condition, and degree of disability. You don't want to keep a fox in an aquarium, a fawn in a cat kennel, or several critters crammed into any one container. You will need to have a variety of clean, intact, and varied sizes and types of containers available for your critters. When I started out I took out cheap ads in the local thrift newspapers to get free aquariums, pet kennels, and rabbit hutches. I went to the local dollar store to purchase the little plastic containers with the holes in them and a variety of brushes, dishes, and other items.

You will probably find you will have to make modifications to your container. What I do is place good-quality mesh over the large holes of my containers so nobody gets in our out. This way nobody gets their head or other body part caught in a hole. This also reduces stress. I flip my pet kennels upside down and put a handle on the top, so the birds can benefit from darkness at their face level but have air at their foot level, allowing me to mist their feet with water from a spray bottle during hot weather. I began doing this after noticing birds would toodle over to their water dishes and cool off by standing in them. Make sure your aquarium has a fitted top; don't underestimate the prowess of a determined escapee! If a small critter gets loose in your house, you may never see it again!

I am very careful with my food and water dishes. I like for the animal to get what they need without falling in. An animal can drown in a teeny tiny water dish. I like to use lids from the gallon water jugs, and lids from a variety of jars for water and food dishes. I like to use sturdy plastic plant saucers in every size, from small to huge, for water dishes. I find this allows the animal to bathe and drink without falling in and drowning. Frisbees are a great water dish/food dish/bath for some birds and other critters. And remember, eating out of a dish is foreign to most animals. Sometimes they won't eat unless the food ISN'T in a dish. And remember that some water birds will eat only if their food is in their water. I don't use side-mounted water bottles for mammals; after all, they won't be seeing too many of those once they're free.

What about cage furniture for your critters? Depending on the animal, it can be as simple as a cardboard paper towel tube, a pile of hay, a bark-covered log, or a big flannel pillowcase. Some mammals enjoy animal-safe toys for exercise and stimulation. Some animals get a huge kick out of playing with their food. Some like ladders and/or elaborate jungle gyms for physical therapy. Again, ask your sponsor and other rehabbers what works for them. Rehabbers are very resourceful people that come up with great ideas on what works, usually born of necessity and unavailability of items we need.

One thing I hope you will keep in mind is choice. Every animal should have a choice about comfort. A wire-bottomed enclosure can hurt sensitive paws and feet. A surface that is too soft can hurt tough raptor feet. An animal should be able to move toward or away from a heat source in an enclosure. An animal should be able to enjoy the sun or go rest in the shade. A bird should have the opportunity to bathe in a clean dish or roll around on a comfy surface. Some mammals like to dig, and when they're ready to dig, they should be allowed to dig. Same goes for climbers, swimmers, runners, and fliers; I think you're getting the picture. Once they're ready, an animal needs the opportunity to play, groom themselves, interact with others, and heal.

I have to talk about feet again. An animal that spends the majority of its time on its feet, like a bird, needs a choice of a variety of surfaces to rest on to keep their feet healthy, otherwise they could develop bumble foot, which can be a nasty problem and one they may not recover from. I don't recommend smooth dowels or other smooth, slick surfaces like that for perching. I recommend a branch with bark AND a soft surface AND if you can, a chunk of sod. CHOICES, remember?

Lets' talk about transport containers if you're in a pinch. My favorite is a cardboard box with small ventilation holes poked in it and the lid taped securely shut. Why? It's SOO not glamorous but in my opinion, highly effective.

We talked about stress. With many birds and mammals, once you place them in that box with a towel or a piece of carpet on the bottom so they're not slipping and sliding around, and once they're in the dark, their stress level tends to drop. Don't use a towel with holes, strings, or loops. I like carpet because I can get big pieces donated from carpet stores. I cut the carpet to fit my kennels and then throw them away when I'm done. Astroturf is another good, non-skid surface for feet. Also, my favorite source of heat in a container is a sand-filled disc, available at pet supply and rehab supply places. This is a flat disc that you heat up in your microwave. It won't roll around in the container, in the car, and squish your critter. Be sure you place the towel or carpet OVER the disc so the critter doesn't get burned and be sure the critter can get away from the heat if it needs to. I don't like grass, leaves, branches, or other objects in transport containers because I worry someone might fall off of it or onto it, or otherwise have an accident. And the cardboard, in my opinion, is great because it de-stresses the animal, keeps them safe during the transport, and doesn't ruin feathers and fur, like wire cages can. And cardboard you can dispose of. Once you've had enough of your nice expensive kennels disappear you'll probably come to love the cardboard box as much as I do!

When transporting live animals, make sure they are very secure. If a critter gets out in your car while you're driving and disappears, you might never see it again. You probably don't want rodents loose in there, chewing upholstery and wires. You don't want an animal bailing out the car window while you're driving or flapping in your face while you're trying to see and drive.

CLEANING UP YOUR ACT

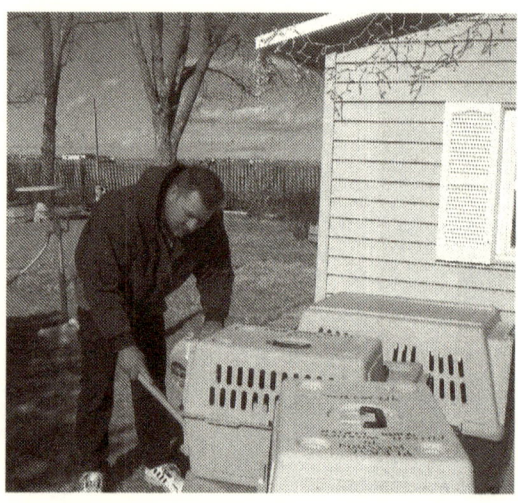

Keeping your facility-your house-clean as a home-based rehabber can be quite a challenge. And you'd be amazed how messy some critters are!

Healthy animals living free keep themselves pretty clean. Birds poop off the side of the nest and away from themselves to keep the nest and their body clean. Mammals poop away from where they eat and sleep. I'm not sure but I think geese poop just about everywhere!

An animal in rehab (in captivity) doesn't have the opportunity to keep itself as clean as it would outside in nature. So it is our job to keep them as clean as we can. Sometimes this means cleaning up the animal and always this means cleaning up the animals' containers and supplies.

We need to clean the containers, bedding, dishes, and equipment. Keep ease of cleaning in mind when you're collecting supplies. If you find yourself with a lot of critters, quick and efficient clean-up is an art. If you care for babies, plan on changing their bedding and sometimes even those containers at least every time you feed them.

I prefer to use whatever I can that is disposable. This includes paper cups for formula, paper plates for food prep, and disposable dairy soakers that I buy from the grocery stores. These are padded on one side and plastic on the other, and are not perfumed like pet pads. I purchase cheap paper towels by the case, and unscented, un-dyed tissue. I use brushes from the dollar store and dispose of them when I change out the container or cage.

It is important not to mix your people dishes with your animal dishes for cleaning. Same goes for linens and just about everything else. Avoid cross-contamination between your stuff and your animal stuff, and between the different animal items themselves, as much as you possibly can.

As far as cleaning materials, everyone has their own idea on what works best for them. Personally, for cleaning up after birds, I wear a disposable mask because birds are very dusty and breathing in too much bird dust might cause respiratory problems. I also wear disposable gloves for cleaning up after the critters. Maybe I should buy stock in disposable gloves …

Sometimes hot water and vinegar is enough to clean up that mess. There are times you'll need to use bleach. Remember that bleach is very corrosive. There are times you might use Nolvasan. When I need regular soap I use biodegradable, environmentally safe products. My favorite soap is a vegetable-based, all-purpose product from the health food store. Instead of chemical-laden, perfumed dryer sheets I use liquid fabric softener from the health food store.

Some of your equipment might need to be boiled or if you lucky enough to have one, autoclaved. Maybe you're lucky enough to have a pressure washer!

I keep gavage tubes in a variety of sizes on hand and also lots of needle-less syringes in a variety of sizes, in particular, the 1 mL size. If I have lots of baby birds I'm feeding, I use these syringes to feed the babies but dispose of them when I'm done, and use new syringes for the next round. I go through an incredible amount of syringes this way but that's okay with me. I don't have time to sterilize the syringes each time I use them. I don't use sticks or stirrers, or anything that's sharp on the end to feed animals. I don't want to risk perforation. I don't use the same syringe to feed all the babies, to avoid cross-contamination.

Cleaning your outdoor facilities can be just as much fun as cleaning your indoor facilities. I keep a cleaning brush from the dollar store and a shovel and rake at each cage for routine cleaning. When I change out the cages to make room for a new animal, the brush is disposed of and replaced with a new one. The rakes and shovels are cleaned very thoroughly.

When changing out the cages I also clean the dirt or if need be, I replace it altogether. This, I feel, is particularly important for mammals. I wear gloves and a mask to clean the outdoor cages, and begin cleaning by hosing down the entire cage, from top to bottom, to lower the airborne particles. I don't want to inhale that junk. I get my bleach and pressure sprayer, and bleach the entire cage from top to bottom, including the dirt.

I check the cage "furniture" for damage and for mold. If anything in the cage is moldy it is disposed of and replaced-thank goodness for young people building these items as volunteer projects! I sure go through a lot of nest boxes and ladders. I don't use straw because it has been a problem here with mold. I use fresh hay for bedding if I need to, and keep it dry and fresh.

My personal preference is keeping all items, including dishes and linens, very separate and apart from everything else. I don't like the idea of mixing raccoon items with items for other animals, and especially items used for people. I also feel that raccoon kennels, containers, and cages should contain only raccoons, always and forever, and nothing else.

YOUR OUTDOOR PRERELEASE ENCLOSURE

If you live in the city limits, you likely won't be able to build an aviary or outdoor enclosure in your back yard due to zoning. Find out before building or it could cost you.

If you are allowed to build an outdoor enclosure, that can be a very good thing. A few things to keep in mind are size, construction, predator-proofing, and cost.

When I was starting out my money was very limited, just like now! I used my income tax refund to build my first cage. Then I was awarded a small grant to build another. Sometimes people donated stuff they couldn't use and I built cages out of them. Many years later I was awarded larger grants to build bigger and better enclosures. Do the best you can with what you have.

If you're going to spend the money on an outdoor enclosure, please do it as best you can. Don't go sloppy, or you could be sorry. There's nothing worse than going outside one morning to find your critter has "self-released" or that a predator has been in your cage and killed everything inside. Raccoons (from the inside and from the outside) can open just about anything. They will bend wire, chew wire, and pull sleeping birds through the little holes in the wire to eat them, piece by piece. They will go underneath a wire-bottomed rabbit hutch and chew the feet off those rabbits. If you're going to have an outdoor enclosure in bear or mountain lion territory, more power to you! You might need to bring your animals AND their food indoors overnight. Weasels and snakes can get in your cages, too. Foxes and coyotes are good diggers, and you don't want them digging in our out.

I'll tell you about my cages and maybe some of these ideas will work for you. I presently have 15 cages outside, from very small to very large, for animals of varying sizes and disabilities. Animals are "graduated" from small cages to larger afte their time indoors, ultimately ending up in the largest cages prior to release.

Most of my outdoor enclosures are made from half-by-one-inch welded wire, anc wired top, bottom, and sides. The floors are wired to the sides and the sides to the top. I place a few inches of good dirt on the floors to allow the vegetation to grow through as well as for the animals' feet to be comfortable. My cages are rectangle with double doors for security. The sides and tops of both ends are covered fo shade and shelter, and the middle part of the roof is left open for sun, stars, anc rain. I am on a very limited budget so for visual barriers and privacy I use viny garden lattice and plywood, applied on the inside, and available from home improvement stores. The cages are wired with the sharp edges directed outside of the cages. Inside the cages are a variety of perches, platforms, ladders, logs, and nest boxes, depending on what critter is in there. The water bird cage has a pond and pools in the summertime.

I don't recommend using netting. We don't want our animals getting hung in there.

You can find ideas by visiting other rehabbers and rehab facilities to see what good ideas they have. Talk to them and ask them if they could do anything different, what that would be and why?

WHAT DO I FEED THEM?

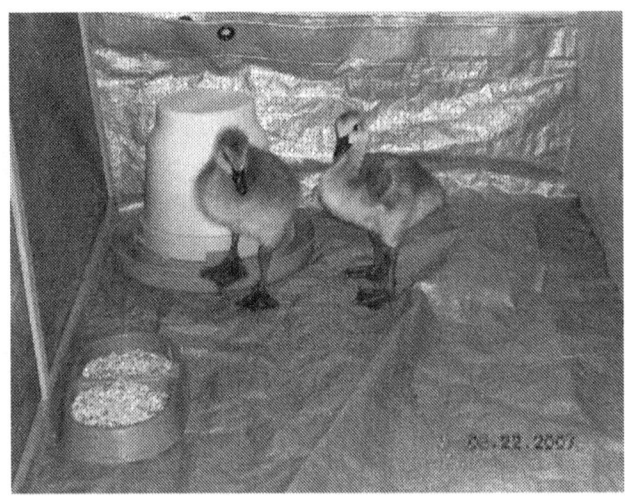

Goslings.

This can be a very hot topic among rehabbers. I'm going to discuss only what works for me and if you like to, feel free to poll other rehabbers to see what works for them.

I make sure water is always available to all of my animals. I've been told there's no need to provide a water dish for raptors, as they don't drink from dishes. Remember our talk about choices? I can tell you from my own experience that not only do raptors absolutely, positively drink from water dishes if they're offered the opportunity but they also enjoy a nice bath as well. Some raptors (kites) enjoy playing with their food in their water dish. Make sure ALL of your animals have fresh water every single day.

I am a firm believer in a natural diet for these wild birds and animals. I believe it is what is best for them to be healthy and successful upon release. I believe a natural diet is a whole diet and that supplements are therefore not usually necessary. I believe we should feed wild animals the food that they can recognize and find once they're released. If you are too squeamish to feed your animals properly, this isn't the kind of work for you. If you have moral and ethical dilemmas regarding predator/prey feeding issues, this might not be the work or right animal species for you. There is no substitute for a proper diet and if the animal is deprived of it, they will suffer later on.

You will be amazed at how expensive it can be to feed wild birds and animals. You might need a variety of formulas, fruits, vegetables, nuts, seeds, grains, fish and crustaceans, bugs and meat, grasses and hays, among other items, for your animals. By meat, I don't mean chemically-treated or flavor-treated meats from the grocery store. By meat I mean rodents, poultry, fish, and bugs you will get from a specialty vendor. You might have to feed live food to your predators. You will probably have plenty of food prep to get used to, depending on the disabilities of your animals.

Please don't skimp on the food! Make the effort to provide them with what they need. You might be out there in your nightie catching bugs in your butterfly net or outside in your jammies swatting flies. You might be sloshing around at the edge of a pond gathering green goodies for your water birds. You might be trapping rodents in your barn for your predators or setting up light bulbs, sheets, and buckets of water to catch moths. You might be wiping out the local feeder fish supply or worm supply at the pet stores. If you have time to raise meat for your critters, more power to you. Beware; this can be a full-time job.

Consider diet in relation to time of year. If your critter is in rehab for a while, research the winter/spring/summer/fall diet as in some birds and mammals their diet changes with the seasons. Accommodate those differences.

Another note. Please be very, very careful about where your food comes from. Don't accept donated dog food or other food that's overrun with rodents and rodent poop or maggots. Don't accept rodents for your predator unless you know for certain they haven't ingested poison. Don't use nasty old meat. Sometimes breeders will offer donated animals for you to feed your predators. You need to be very certain these animals haven't been chemically euthanized or otherwise chemically treated. Sometimes I'll get a call after the prairie dog colony has been wiped out, asking if I will take the dead dogs to feed my predators. I always say No. Remember that the animals in our care deserve the best we can give them. You will likely need to do research and/or ask other rehabbers for help when determining what to feed your critters. Find out what the natural diet for that animal is as it pertains to your location and time of year.

Regarding babies. There are several commercial formulas out there for mammals and birds. Find one or a combination of them that works for you.

Keep in mind that some baby mammals can't go to the bathroom by themselves at a certain age. You will need to help those babies by stimulating them to go. The mother will lick the area to facilitate urination and defecation. I use a very wet, warm tissue in a rapid motion to get the babies going, and this usually needs to be done before and/or after each feeding. Once the babies are eliminating on their own, you don't need to help them anymore. Just make sure they're eliminating regularly.

Your local and/or online **health food store** can be a very valuable resource for a variety of specialty and hard-to-find items such as unique organic produce items, dried plants and fruits, nuts and seeds, earth—and animal-friendly cleaning products, and homeopathic and plant extract products.

HOW DO I FEED THEM?

Sometimes we get animals in rehab that simply cannot feed themselves. So we need to help them.

This isn't a medical how-to book so I'll give a very, very broad overview.

Don't stuff food down a cold animal. Don't stuff food down a dehydrated animal. Don't stuff food down an animal that can't swallow or has a plaque or other obstruction in its mouth or throat. If your vet/sponsor/other rehabber has time, ask them to show you how to look for the signs of dehydration, hyper—or hypothermia, obstruction, or other obstacles to feeding your critter.

Before feeding animals, they need to be warmed up, hydrated, free of obstructions, and calm. Your vet/sponsor/other rehabber can help you with these processes. We all have the impulse to feed and/or water an animal but that can be what pushes them over the edge. Take a deep breath, calm down, step back, and see what needs to be done before feeding. If I am getting an animal from a vet, I ask if they have time to rehydrate the animal before I pick it up. That helps jump-start the process.

About feeding technique. There is eye-dropper feeding, syringe-feeding, gavage (tube) feeding, hand-feeding. Learn the various feeding techniques to try to avoid aspirating or choking your animal. Tube-feeding is a technique that I found very scary at first (in part because I made a dead pigeon bleed.) But once you have this technique down, you'll sure be glad you learned it to feed pigeons and doves, sick water birds (yummy-blended up fish in a tube!) and other sick birds and animals. Gavage can also be a good route for oral hydration, getting the liquid into the GI system better. Feeding liquids can create the possibility of aspiration, which can be fatal. Proper feeding technique is critical.

Subcutaneous fluid administration is something I find helpful also. Ask your vet/sponsor/rehabber to teach you how to do this if you're interested.

Be sure to prepare the food correctly to feed the animals. You might need to heat it up, grind it up, chop it up, blend it up, pulverize it, or whatever.

And be sure to stick to a feeding schedule. Baby birds and mammals in particular will suffer if fed improper food and aren't fed on a regular feeding schedule.

ABOUT MEDICINE

Sometimes the vet will send you home with an antibiotic or some form of medical treatment. Sometimes this is helpful, sometimes you collect a lot of antibiotic that you simply don't need because the animal has no infection. Dispose of medicine responsibly and ask your veterinarian to help you with this. Again, I find the less chemical interference, the better. However, there are times an animal needs the drug.

If your animal needs medication, sometimes it can be administered orally via placing it in their food (works well with raptors and critters that will eat whole rodents.) Sometimes you can grind it into a powder and place it in some applesauce. Sometimes you will have it in a liquid form and can squirt a little bit very carefully into a mouth. Sometimes you will apply medicine to skin and/or eyes.

And sometimes you'll just have to bite the bullet and give an injection. You might want to learn about medicine administration from your vet/sponsor/other rehabber.

TO DEBUG OR NOT TO DEBUG?

Again, this is subjective and each rehabber has his or her own opinion, based on a variety of reasons, of why they do or do not debug their critters. Again I'm just telling you what works for me.

I find that most of the time in birds, the mites tend to be species-specific and not much of a threat to the bird's health. In a healthier bird, the mites usually stay on the bird. But in a bird that is sick and weak, and has been down for a while, they seem to carry a larger load of mites that can run on to you. This can freak you out a little if it hasn't happened to you before. It stands to reason the mites can't be a good thing for a bird in this condition. I use an over-the-counter preparation to get rid of the mites.

Something else I find in birds, in particular doves, pigeons, and the raptors that eat them, is Trichomonas. A veterinarian can swab the bird orally and show you the organism. If you have a good microscope and know what to look for you can do it yourself. Trichomonas can cause serious problems for birds, including starvation due to obstruction by the plaque that forms in their oropharynx, sometimes obscuring the throat.

One thing about trich I would like to share with you. When I was new, I was told to look in the beak and if the bird had trich, I would see the plaque. And yes, I have had birds where I was easily able to see the plaque. But the bird can be loaded with trich and you'll never see it by looking in the beak. The organism can be lodged around the animal's internal organs and in the sinuses, too. If you see the plaque, I don't recommend pulling it out or off. You could cause pain and bleeding. Treated properly and with a little bit of time, the plaque should slough off by itself.

And that's the good thing about trich; it can be treated. Just know that the bird can contract it again after release. What I do at my facility is prophylactically treat for trich every pigeon, dove, and bird-eating raptor that comes through my door. Some rehabbers don't. Some do. It's up to the rehabber. To me it's just the logical thing to do; when these birds seem so susceptible to trich and that I've seen so many with it, and the same in the predators that eat them. Again, up to the rehabber.

Lice, fleas, and ticks. Personally, I don't bring any mammal into my facility (my house) without treating it first with an over-the-counter parasite preparation. That's just how I do it. Find a preparation that works for you or if you're lucky, maybe the vet will handle that for you before you pick up that animal.

Worms. Roundworms, tapeworms; worms, worms, worms! Some rehabbers de-worm, some don't. Mammals can carry worms and that's just a fact of life. Again, personally I de-worm mine or ask that they be de-wormed before coming to my facility. Because of the roundworm specific to raccoons, I don't rehab raccoons and I don't accept donated items that have had raccoons in them. You can do some research on the raccoon roundworm if you like. Plenty of rehabbers provide care to raccoons but I'm not one of them.

RELEASE PREPARATION

We want to set our wildlife up for success. We want to release them healthy, strong, weather-proof, and properly socialized. We want to release them in the right place at the right time. I feel the release is every bit as important as the rehab.

Maybe you have outdoor release facilities in which to do the prerelease conditioning of your critter. Maybe you don't, and will turn them over to another licensed rehabber for prerelease training in their outdoor enclosures. Whichever the case, understand that these animals shouldn't go from your house to freedom without prerelease training.

Familiarize yourself with and learn as much as you can about release criteria. In Colorado the animal must have all of its parts; both wings, both/all legs, both eyes, the tail, etc. and all of these parts must be in 100% working condition. Otherwise the law requires the animal be euthanized, with some exceptions made for raptors that you can learn about some time. Currently in Colorado there is no permanent sanctuary for native-born, nonreleaseable wildlife.

We need to know if the animal is socialized to its own kind or are is it going to be out there chasing people around for food? Can digging animals dig? Can birds fly and land properly? Can squirrels climb properly? Is the animal acclimated to weather and are the wings/fur waterproof? Is this animal prepared to recognize and find food? Does this animal recognize a predator? Is this animal tame or imprinted? If so, this animal is not releaseable.

Research your release site and time! I'm guessing as newbies we've all had the horrific experience taking lots of time, energy, and money caring for a bird that we had all ready for release in its outdoor flight cage. Then we open that cage door and here's the magical moment; freedom! Your little finch flies toward the pine tree and right in front of your eyes is snatched from midair by the opportunistic hawk, and eaten on your front porch. This experience is enough to make some rehabbers quit rehabbing. But it can be a very important lesson.

I've learned that keeping songbirds in outdoor enclosures seems to draw the resident raptor population. Therefore releasing songbirds (and cottontails) is tricky for me. I no longer release the majority of my songbirds in my yard, like I used to do. There's nothing worse than witnessing your bird that you've had since a pink, naked, eyes-closed critter being carried off into the sunset by a predator.

Release your animals during the right time of day. Nocturnal animals, such as nighttime owls and bats, shouldn't be released during the afternoon. You wouldn't want to release a songbird at nighttime.

Research your release site. Ideally your animal should go back where it came from. If this isn't possible due to the area being undesirable or if the birds in that area have migrated, you need to find out where the migratory population of that bird is and get permission to release it there. Watch the extended weather forecast and look for a spell of good weather.

Sometimes you might need to do a soft release, which is possible if you have critters of the same species in your yard and wish to give them a few days to join the flock.

Obtain permission from a property owner before releasing animals on their property.

QUALITY OF LIFE AND MAKING THE HARD DECISIONS

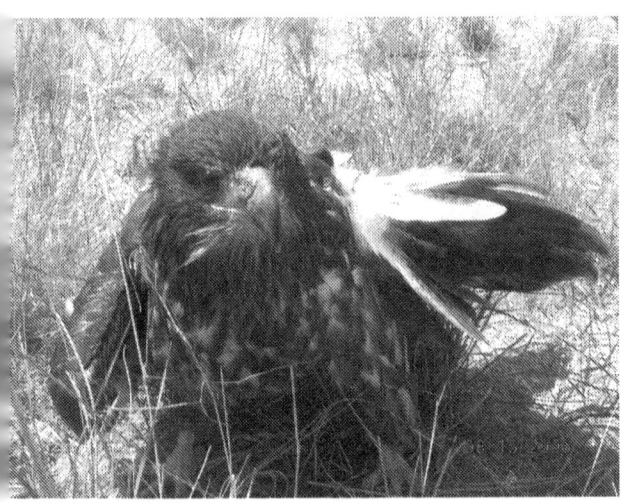

Immature bald eagle.

Quality of life is everything. In wildlife rehabilitation, you will have to make some very tough decisions regarding quality of life and euthanasia. It gets a little bit easier with time and experience but really, I'm still left with the same feeling after sending a critter to the vet for chemical release.

With time and experience we are better able to identify if an animal is enjoying any quality of life. Is the critter pain-free, eating and taking care of itself? Or is it huddled up in a ball in the corner, not eating? Is it self-destructive? Has it given up on life?

An adult animal that has lived its life free, I think, has a much harder time adjusting to captivity than a baby that has nothing to compare it to. That's why I feel it is so important that we do everything we can to make that animal comfortable by providing a stress-free, stimulating environment; by providing natural food and an opportunity to enjoy some sunshine and fresh air if they're able to.

Making the life-or-death decision is easier if the animal is in obvious pain. It is not so easy a decision when the animal has some good days and some bad days. Even after all this time, I still second-guess euthanasia. Sometimes I wonder if I should have done it sooner. Sometimes I wonder if I should have given the animal more time. It's gut-wrenching when you have an animal with spirit that obviously is never going to meet release criteria that you know you have to have euthanized.

I've experienced days and weeks when I wonder why I do this work. It can be so depressing. I wonder if it really matters. I wonder if anyone cares. I think how nice it would be to not have the crushing responsibility. I eat a pound of chocolate and go to bed.

Later on I realize there are many others right now that need me. If I give up, I can't help them. I realize that it's amazing, when I think about it, that any of these animals that end up in rehab make it at all. I realize I am so very lucky for the beautiful release days.

With time I think we all become better at determining quality of life. It means everything.

OH, HAPPY RELEASE DAY!

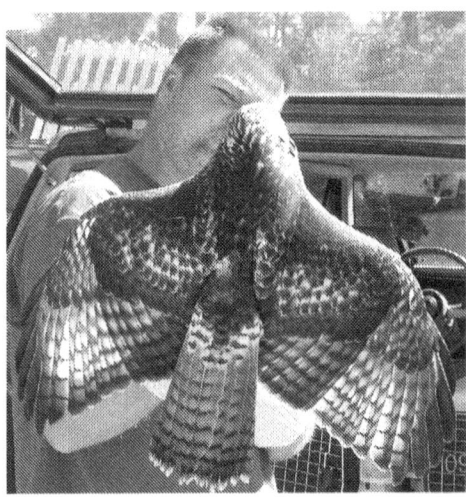

Red-tailed hawk.

Oh, this is so exciting! Remember what that critter looked like when he came to rehab? Maybe he was naked and pink with eyes still closed. Maybe he came after a car hit with a broken leg. Maybe he came to rehab convulsing from poison. Maybe he came to rehab temporarily blind and paralyzed after colliding with a car or window. Maybe he showed up tangled in fishing line with a monster of a hook in his gullet and a belly full of lead. Maybe he showed up dehydrated and starving after being pulled out of a dumpster. Whatever the case, look how good he looks now!

All of your hard work has paid off; the time, the paperwork, the sleepless nights, the phone calls … Perhaps you'd like to invite the animal's finder to the release. This is what I do if I can, and this shows the animal finder that they did the right thing by stopping to pick up that animal and find help. It shows the animal finder that they did the right thing by turning it over to someone that could care for it. I feel it's a good outreach effort and creates a connection between the animal and the finder. You might find that the release is a very emotional (in a good way) moment for that person and means a lot to them. Again I have to repeat myself by saying that I feel the work we do is just as much about helping people as it is about helping the animals. Snatching the animal away from a concerned member of the community and not returning their phone calls to see how their animal is doesn't give that person a good feeling about wildlife rehabbers. Be nice. Release is another opportunity to share the experience with the person that without you wouldn't be doing wildlife rehab in the first place.

Now that you're ready for release I recommend packing up you camera, carefully loading up your critter, and heading off to do your release.

I've learned over the years that not all releases are movie-perfect. Sometimes they don't want to come out of their kennel. Sometimes they don't soar overhead but sit on the ground for a while to get their bearings. Usually they head the opposite direction of where your camera is pointed. Releases can be unpredictable and that's okay. Sometimes they do bound off into the forest. Sometimes they do soar overhead. I've had a few releases that were frankly unspectacular but these are animals and animals can be unpredictable. I always allow the animal finder to get a quick picture or two before the animal is released.

After your release you can pack up your supplies, get back in your car, take a deep breath and let it out, and celebrate this joyous occasion. The release, in my opinion, is what wildlife rehab is all about.

MY THOUGHTS ON BABY BIRDS

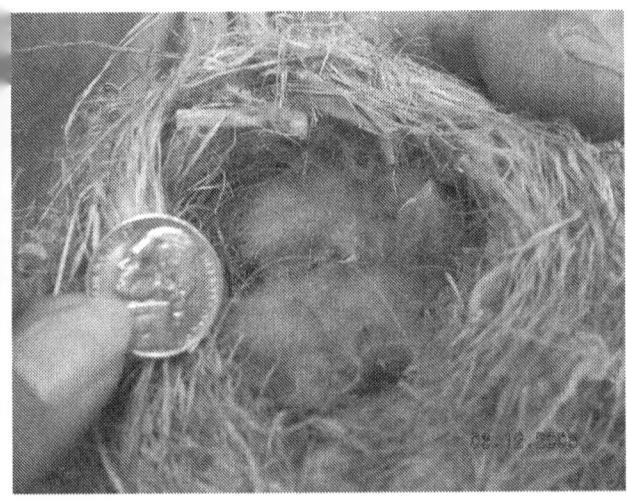

Yep, people will bring you lots of these!

I've already mentioned the great need for good baby bird rehabbers in Colorado. I imagine it's true in every state. If you're not careful you can find yourself with 100+ in the space of a day. Baby birds have a very stringent feeding schedule and it can run you ragged, with some species requiring feedings every 15 minutes or so, from sunup to sundown.

Baby birds have different means of being fed by the adults. Some baby birds gape for you, which makes feeding them a whole lot easier. Some baby birds like pigeons and doves won't gape for you at all, which means there's a very real possibility you will want to learn gavage (tube) feeding technique, which allows you feed the proper amount, keeping it warm, very quickly. If you are not comfortable with tube feeding then syringe feeding might work for you but it's messy and can take longer, and you'll need to make sure your formula is warm. Never feed cold food or formula to any animal, at any time. Some baby birds come out of their shell eating on their own and that makes your life a lot easier. Just be sure you're providing the proper food and the heat lamp. Some babies need their food chopped up into little juicy pieces and will eat them on their own if you wiggle the food around a little bit.

Baby birds have different nutritional needs. Some are insect-eaters, some seed-eaters, some meat-eaters, and some fish-and crustacean-eaters. You could very well be spending a large part of your morning preparing the foods for the variety of birds you will be feeding. There are commercial hand-feeding baby bird formulas out there. Some rehabbers like them and some don't. Find what works for you. What I like to do is take a basic commercial formula and modify it. Don't feed these commercial corn-based formulas to baby raptors.

- Be prepared for the fact that you will be shelling out a lot of money to feed babies the appropriate food. It's just something that you must do. Know your limitations!

- Raptors are carnivores and need whole foods, prepared accordingly. Don't imprint your raptors; it is illegal. If you don't have a foster raptor I recommend sending the baby to a facility that does, in the best interest of the bird.

- Baby water birds, particularly ducklings and goslings, shouldn't be placed in water while still downy as they may not be able to maintain their body temperatures. I give them a poultry waterer or a shallow dish so they can drink without immersing themselves. I provide a heat lamp for them. It is very important that their heat source comes from above, not a heating pad. I feed them commercial poultry pellets and plenty of green produce items. I keep their food right near the water, as they seem to enjoy mixing them all together and making a big, stinky mess! They will run back and forth from the water and food to the heat lamp, which is why I keep them at opposite ends of the container.

- Baby hummingbirds. I use a commercial formula by Nekton for hummingbirds, supplemented with freeze-dried insects.

- Weaning finches and others. My trick is organic, unsweetened applesauce with the weaning food mixed in and the applesauce being made less and less until the bird is eating what it's supposed to be.

- Variety of foods. Remember we talked about choices. What I do is offer a veritable buffet for all of my songbirds and corvids. I offer nuts, seeds, grains, fruits, vegetables, and meats. They will find what they like and what they need, and you know they are eating well.

- For woodpeckers. Use logs with bark on them. Drill some holes, fill with goodies like wax worms or peanut butter. They like moving food (worms and ants) and can eat a LOT. They like fruits (watermelon, berries, etc.) and these foods will attract ants and other moving bugs they like.

- Watermelon is something I keep in my 'fridge all day, every day, each and every day of the year. I use it as a tool to get a young bird to wean or a resistant bird to self-feed, and then to eat what it is supposed to eat. I use it as a source of fluids for an animal that can't drink, to supplement the fluids I'm giving the other ways. For me it is a wonderful item that makes life easier for everyone. However, remember, just like everything else, it's never the ONLY thing I offer a critter, just a small part.

- Robins. While the babies are still young (but feathered) I take a dishpan or similar container, fill it with clean dirt and worms and other bugs, and let the robins have their fun! They need to find bugs before release and this seems to help. That way once they're outside in prerelease they have a head start. I definitely do NOT recommend stuffing your baby robins full of night crawlers, as so many people want to do. Night crawlers aren't their entire diet and can make the robin sick with gapeworm. Remember-VARIETY. Robins eat a variety of insects as well as worms and fruits.

- Mealworms and wax worms. Again, opinions on the subject of feeding worms like these to baby and compromised birds varies from rehabber to rehabber. Personally, I feed mealworms only if they're small and with the heads removed. I was bitten by a mealworm once and it was nasty. It made me wonder if the worm chews inside the baby bird. Also mealworms seem hard and dry to me. I prefer wax worms. They are plump, soft, and full of moisture. The birds seem to tolerate them quite well. I supplement the mix of worms and bugs for insect-eaters with the bugs I catch outside as well and the freeze-dried insects available at the pet stores. Variety!

- Be very, very careful that your babies don't imprint on you.

- Stacking babies, fighting babies, nest behavior. Keep a close eye out for stacking babies that pile up on top of each other, smothering the ones on the bottom. Keep an eye out for fighting babies, too. Separate them as needed.

BUNNIES; BABIES AND OTHERWISE

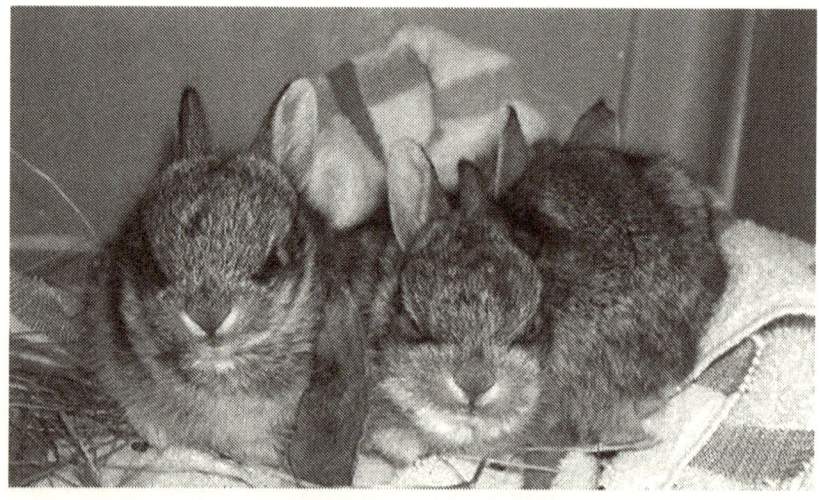

Baby bunnies can break your heart!

I could tell you I'm brimming with success regarding baby cottontail and jackrabbit rehab. That would be a big, fat lie. I will tell you that I have terrible, terrible luck with neonate cottontails. I lose almost every single one. I have tried every formula and combination of formulas. I have tried every old wives' tale formula. I have tried every latest new food items for the neonates. I've tried every feeding technique. The outcome is still the same; I lose just about every single one of those neonate cottontails. I don't even take them into rehab here anymore. It's just too depressing. Some rehabbers relay amazing success statistics of their neonates. Hooray to you, I'll send the neonate bunnies to you and good luck! Personally, I feel there's something they need from their mother and when they come to rehab they either have it or they don't. And there's nothing we can substitute it with. Before you get all excited, yes, I have tried colostrum, acidophilus, yogurt, goat's milk, commercial formulas, and on and on and on. Nothing works for me. Not even "bunny poop tea."

It's always the same for me. I feed them, stimulate them (baby mammals need to be stimulated to urinate and defecate) and manage to keep them alive for several days, and sometimes even to weaning. I lose them during weaning. I get up one morning and find they have died. I've never had the nasty diarrhea in my cottontails or any of the other seemingly endless problems like that I read and hear so much about. They look great, begin eating on their own, and then die. I just can't even believe it.

I have spoken with rehabbers all over the Nation. I have spoken with rabbit breeders. None of these people have anything to offer me that helps.

I will tell you that I have pretty good luck with rabbits that come to me with their eyes opened and weaned. I do pretty well with car-hit rabbits, degloved rabbits, and rabbits with other injuries. I think the luck has plenty to do with the stress-free, quiet environment. It also helps if you have another cottontail in rehab, as rabbits are pretty social and seem to derive comfort from knowing they're not all alone.

In my experience with rabbits it seems that less is more. Again, I beg you, don't drown yourself in perfume or use other stinky, smelly, perfumed air fresheners, candles, incense, dryer sheets, and things like, and don't smoke when working with rabbits (and other mammals, for that matter.) Rabbits in particular seem sensitive to smells-maybe because they're on the bottom of the food chain and rely on smell in regard to predators?

Rabbits seem easily stressed by noise (I do believe we've covered this) and handling. A rabbit, even a baby, can be an amazing jumper and a pretty quick runner. You don't want a rabbit jumping out of your hands and breaking its back or running under your entertainment center.

In my experience, less is more with regard to working with wild rabbits and jacks. Less chemical treatment seems to be a good thing. I never, ever give a rabbit an antibiotic unless I see or smell an infection. I never, ever allow that rabbit to be given steroids. If a rabbit has lacerations or puncture wounds, I use flower-extract gels (not creams) and homeopathic remedies instead of chemically-prepared solutions. They seem to benefit from this. I rarely have the vet suture rabbit skin, as this seems to create more problems than it solves because as the rabbit moves, the skin will continue to tear. Rabbits have very fragile skin.

Rabbits have rather complex digestive systems. I don't recommend a diet that is too rich or too complex. Personally, I don't use alfalfa hay at all for my bunnies, whether they are my rehab rabbits or my domestic rabbits. I keep fresh timothy hay available at all times for all of the rabbits. I prefer to order orchard grasses, timothy pellets, and critical care rabbit formula from a supplier out of state. I want hay and grass that is free of mold. I want pelleted food that is cold-processed and fresh, green, and smells like what it is-grass and hay. I don't want old food that is brown or gray and has turned to dust. I don't want food that has junk in it.

If you screw up your rabbit's digestive system, you may not ever get it back to normal.

Bunnies are (like me) carbohydrate fiends. My domestic rabbits will just about stand on their heads and do cartwheels for a goody. Wild rabbits are no different. I don't give them a lot of junk. I give them all the same thing; the good hay, the good pellets, and fresh greens. Rabbit pellets can be bought that have little pieces of colored and shaped stuff in it. I don't use that for my rabbits. A rabbit that needs meds or is having difficulty drinking or eating gets fresh watermelon to get him started. That particular rabbit will also have his greens misted with water for extra moisture. Don't give your cottontail or jackrabbit a bunch of garbage in the form of fruits, starchy vegetables, or grains. Give them the carrot tops if you must, but not the carrot! Keep the diet fairly simple. If you're going to offer them fresh grass, make sure it's not full of chemicals.

Bunnies are creatures of routine. They know what time it is no matter what day-light savings time says! Once your wild rabbits know the routine, stick to it. They don't seem to like changes in their routine. A thumping rabbit is telling you something!

If your rabbits can drink, always, always, always make sure they have plenty of fresh, clean water. You'd be surprised how much they drink! Same goes for jack-rabbits, too.

Eating is a social occasion for rabbits. When they can see and hear each other eat, they seem more inspired to eat themselves. The sights and sounds of other rabbits eating seem to have a calming effect on a stressed rabbit.

There comes a time when the baby bunnies might begin to fight. They're still pretty small when this happens so watch carefully and separate as needed.

Bunnies need room to run and play, as well as a place to hide. Please be sure they get this. Bunnies need sunshine for healthy eyes. Bunnies will fight fiercely, too, so don't put a bunch of them together once they are small juvies and older. Once your bunny is in prerelease training in your outdoor cage, he will learn to recognize predators and maybe even get to know the resident bunnies that live free outside.

CRITTER-SITTERS

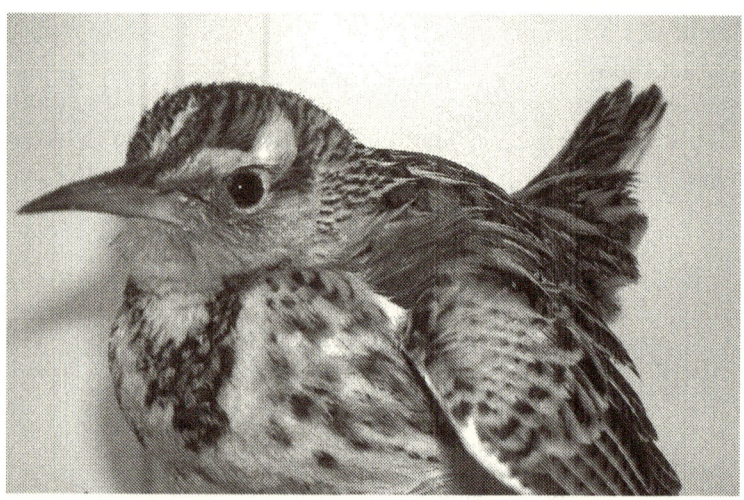

Meadowlark.

There might come a time when you need a critter-sitter for your wildlife. There might come a time when another rehabber asks you to critter-sit for them.

If you ask another rehabber to critter-sit for you, send the food and supplies for the duration if you're able to.

This is a big responsibility and for me, can be a little scary. What happens if their animal dies while under my care? The very idea makes me shudder.

Luck can change and what if? What if this rehabber has had that critter for quite a while, it's doing well, about ready for release, and then it comes to your facility and drops dead? You might be tempted to leave town, never to be heard from again. You might decide to quit rehab. And how in the world do you tell that other rehabber?

Chances are the other rehabber will understand. They might be surprised, they might not. But hopefully we rehabbers understand that things happen and let's ace it, if these animals were completely healthy they wouldn't be in rehab, would hey? They'd be out living life in the wild.

Watching someone else's animals is a big responsibility. We all do the best we can nd hope all goes well. If all doesn't go well, let's not play the blame game. We all now we're going to blame ourselves any, so why make it worse?

Also, if you ask someone else to watch your critter temporarily, be sure it really is emporary and that you take the animal back when you say you will. Don't dump on another rehabber because word travels quickly and other rehabbers won't help ou out next time.

TO RESCUE OR NOT TO RESCUE?

If you have time to rescue AND do rehab, great. You must have more time than do. I will go and do the rescue if I have time and a car. Otherwise, most of the time I rely on volunteers to do the rescue and transport. We have the best, most wonderful DOW volunteer transport team program in Colorado Springs and I rely on them extensively.

As a rehabber you will get calls to rescue animals from the highway, the window well, the chimney, the lake, the sky, and so forth.

You've heard the term "wild goose chase," right? There's a reason it's called that and Heaven help you if you're out there chasing an injured goose around the lake the week before Thanksgiving while the entire middle school is out there on a field trip! The police will show up and inform you you're not allowed to catch your own goose for your holiday dinner. You will have a lot of 'splainin' to do. Keep your permits in your car so you can prove you're legitimate.

A bird that can't run can fly. A bird that can't fly can run. A bird that can't do either can maybe swim. If you're lucky enough that the injured goose is tame enough to come to you for food, you can feed it while someone else sneaks up on it from behind and contains it.

Are you small enough to squeeze into a fox den, full of mud and fleas? Do you have tools in the car for cutting that bird out of barbed wire? How are you going to get from that high-rise roof to the one across the street, while the critter bounces back and forth? You're not seriously going to stand in the middle of I-25 during rush hour, are you? Lucky for me, the Colorado Division of Wildlife has a volunteer transport team that is trained in many aspects of wildlife rescue and handling. And I would never ask them or anyone else to stand on I-25 during any time of the day, dive in the lake, get on the rooftop, to catch a critter!

I'm much older and more tired now than I was a few years ago. If the animal is contained and people are literally standing there watching it to keep track of it, I will go out or ask a volunteer to go out to pick it up. If it's running up and down Nevada Avenue or flying from treetop to treetop, I don't go out or ask anyone else to. If it's dark or stormy, same thing goes. If it's paddling around contentedly on the lake I don't ask anyone to go out onto the lake to try to catch it. I don't have a lot of time, gas is very expensive and I live in the boonies, drive an old car, and no longer go out on wild goose chases. I am considerate of volunteers' time. If it's iffy, I tell the volunteer and let them decide if they want to try or not.

I do NOT ask the Public to do anything risky. Remember the chapter on liability? I might ask them to keep an eye on it until someone gets there if it's safe, like in their yard. I might ask them to throw a box, blanket, or container over it. I don't ever ask them to handle the animal, dive into the lake, or chase that duck up and down Nevada Avenue. Although the DOW volunteers are very well-trained, I don't ask them to do stunt man tricks and I definitely never, ever ask them to act as law enforcement-that's not their job.

I appreciate heroics and sometimes all goes well. Although we are here to help the critters, human life comes first. Let's be safe and responsible.

THE PEOPLE WHO HELP US

I would like to take a moment to talk about working with volunteers, which you will likely be doing if you decide to obtain nonprofit status.

In Colorado Springs, we have the most amazing Division of Wildlife volunteer program. Over the years the DOW transport volunteers have been a team of individuals that I rely on all year long, and they never let me down. The DOW volunteers are the individuals that pick up animals while I'm at work and take them to the vet, and/or to my facility. The DOW volunteers have helped with educational programs, and with facilities expansion and maintenance, and a variety of other projects at my facility. The Colorado Springs DOW volunteers have a gem of a Volunteer Coordinator who is available, personable, and cares a lot about her job and about helping rehabbers and wildlife responsibly. The Volunteer Coordinator interviews and registers volunteers, provides training workshops, and puts together a monthly calendar of volunteer transporter availability. This calendar is a good tool for us rehabbers that rely on the transport team to get wildlife where it needs to go.

The Colorado Springs DOW Volunteer Coordinator also has a team of about 30 or so volunteers that are ready, willing, and able to assist just about anywhere and anytime they are needed. The reason she keeps a consistently great team of volunteers from one year to the next is that she treats people, ALL people, and in particular the volunteers, very well. She says Thank You all the time. She organizes appreciation events and recognition ceremonies. I've noticed over the years it's almost always the same volunteers that are ready to help. I've learned a lot from the Volunteer Coordinator.

Division of Wildlife volunteers are wildlife helpers that are truly dedicated people trained by the DOW. DOW volunteers tend to be experienced in dealing appropriately with the public. They love animals and want to help.

I rely on their help and know that if I abuse the volunteers (and anyone else that helps me) I will be out of luck when I need help, which is often.

I don't ask the volunteers to go out of their way to transport an animal unless they're the unique individual that enjoys a road trip (with expensive prices of gas-yikes!) If it takes me longer on the phone to arrange a transport chain then I prefer to do it that way. This is how I am able to move animals from around the state to where they need to go; a team effort. I try to be considerate of volunteer time. They're busy people just like I am, with jobs, families, medical problems, and so forth. They may be on the calendar for that particular day but when I call they may have done transport already and shouldn't feel they have to do another if they can't. If they are unavailable for some other reason, that's okay; we have a very long list of resources, and I call each and every one until I find someone available for help. I don't berate a volunteer if they can't help me this time.
I don't ask volunteers to break the law. This puts a very kind person in a very nasty situation and it's just plain not fair. Not fair at all.

I don't ask volunteers to act as law enforcement. It's not their job. This is why we have wildlife officers. They can enforce the law, not us and not the volunteers.

I don't ask volunteers to handle animals they are not trained to handle or animals they are uncomfortable with handling.

I don't ask volunteers to handle a situation if I expect it to be dangerous. If a particular volunteer relishes a challenge, then it's up to them to decide if they want this particular call or not. I don't ask volunteers to clamber about rooftops, get out onto the lake, or stand in traffic for a critter. If a situation is particularly tricky I will try to deal with it myself or call the DOW to see if they have resources available.

I try not to ask volunteers to help with a situation that puts them out of their comfort level. This can be tricky because volunteers REALLY want to help and might be hesitant to be straight with me about their feelings on a particular matter. I offer choices and let the volunteer decide if they want to deal with it or not. If not, that's perfectly okay by me. Again, I value human life above animal life and I know we simply can't save them all.

I don't ask volunteers to do anything I wouldn't do.

I appreciate volunteers. I appreciate everything they do. I have learned a lot from volunteers and couldn't possibly have accomplished what I have without their help.

I value the volunteers! I appreciate volunteers by saying Thank You and by not taking advantage of them, or take them for granted. I listen to the people that help me; they have great ideas and more experience in some areas than I do.

TO BE NONPROFIT OR NOT?

A few years into wildlife rehab, I was (still am) seriously behind on bills. Wildlife rehab was costing me thousands of dollars a year, mostly funded by my eensy little paycheck.

My husband was freaking out and we both realized that something had to happen or we would have to drop out of rehab. We simply couldn't afford to pay for it any longer.

So I decided to look into becoming an IRS nonprofit. Boy, was that a scary, expensive, and intimidating process. I had to learn the application process. I recommend a financial person and/or attorney to help you set this up, if you can afford one.

A benefit of obtaining nonprofit status is that when someone makes a donation, they get the benefit of a tax write-off. And believe me, donors will ask about this. Don't misrepresent your status. You'll know you're an IRS nonprofit because you will have a letter from the IRS saying you are. A benefit to becoming a nonprofit is that you can now apply for grants.

A downfall of becoming nonprofit is the paperwork and the other stuff. You will need to incorporate, which means forming a Board of Directors and Officers. You can be small and simple or large and complex; it's up to you. Just make sure the people you choose are all on the same page with the same values and vision of the organization. Make sure these are people that you communicate well with and work well with. The Board and officers should be well-informed and onboard with what the organization is doing. The Board should contribute something to the organization, whether it's expertise, work, or money.

Be sure you know what is required to be nonprofit in your city, county, and State. Get your nonprofit registration, your Articles, and everything else you need. Be timely with your paperwork and make sure it is current. Learn the law regarding raffles, sales tax, etc. if any of these apply to you.

Be prepared for lots of work and paperwork!

DO I BELONG?

You will find there are several wildlife rehab organizations. They can be local and they can be national. They can be helpful, too, in terms of information and resources.

Some rehabbers prefer flying solo, doing their own thing, and that is totally okay. Some rehabbers enjoy more social interaction so joining a club or organization is great for them.

You can choose to become a member of a wildlife rehab organization if you want. You can choose to belong to several. And you can choose not to belong to any. Find out what it costs to join a rehab organization and how becoming a member will benefit you.

Find out if joining more than one organization creates any kind of conflict of interest for you or the organization.

Each organization has its own policies and procedures, so do your homework and ask lots of questions!

THE NUMBERS GAME

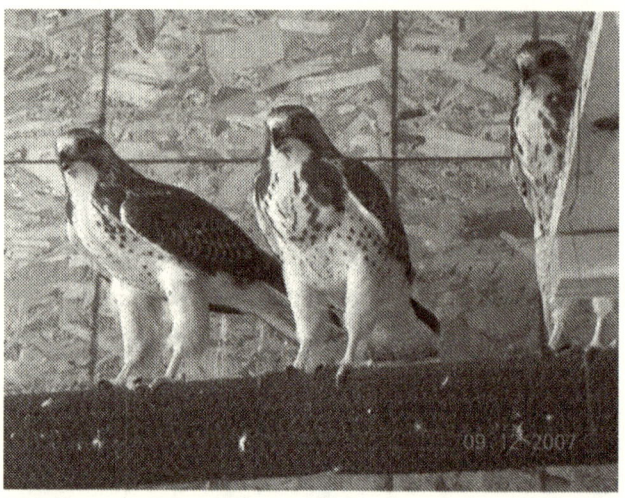

Three young Swainson's hawks.

Numbers can be bent and manipulated in any variety of ways.

For some rehabbers success might be determined by their overall intake numbers; i.e., the more animals taken into rehab the bigger their success rate. Don't take more animals than you can care for to try to pad your numbers and then dump them on other rehabbers. This goes back to knowing your limitations.

One of the ways I determine my success rate in my rehab program is by the percentage of wildlife released or to other program, excluding the DOAs and euthanasias, because obviously they had no chances of being released.

So if you're a rehabber that is able to care for only 10 animals per year and 9 of them were successfully rehabbed to release, you would have a 90% release/success rate. You should be very proud of that. If you take 100 animals into rehab and release 50 of them, you would have a 50% release/success rate, in my book, which still isn't bad at all. If you take 300 animals into rehab and 50 are rehabbed to release, you would want to see what you could do to improve your release rate.

Some rehabbers can provide care only to critical patients in terrible condition that are tough to care for or other rehabbers might not accept into rehab. We can expect that these rehabbers might have lower success rates than those that take only healthy orphaned animals into rehab that we would expect to do much better.

Many things need to be taken into consideration when analyzing the numbers, as they can be very subjective.

I feel that a year when my intake drops is a success, because perhaps that means that my education is reaching the people it needs to and that animals aren't being rushed to rehab when they shouldn't be.

I also determine the success of my rehab program by repeat business. You'd be surprised that in this field that you would even get repeat business, but you do, if you take good care of the people that bring animals to you.

As a very small facility, I feel I have an advantage over larger facilities in that I can give more time-intensive care to the animals that need it. I can do that with one sick bird but I couldn't probably do it if I had 20 sick birds. I think a small facility can be just as beneficial to these animals as a large facility.

AFTERWORD

So do you still think you want to be a rehabber?

Sometimes what you see on TV regarding work with wildlife can seem so interesting and so much fun. Wildlife rehab IS interesting and can be fun, but the reality of the work we all do working out of our homes, the cleaning up and chores; paperwork, phones, etc. can have a significant impact on our quality of life. At my facility very little time is spent in actual hands-on with the animals. Most of the time is spent on chores.

This book is a very broad overview of what rehab can be like and what rehab is like for me. Your experience can be totally different. Everyone is an individual and experience is unique to the individual.

Wildlife rehabilitation is lots of things; rewarding, aggravating, happy and sad, hard work and humor, dirty and enlightening. There are days I feel I am working in a vacuum and that nobody knows or cares about me or these animals. There are days when I wonder if it's all worth it because I'm totally broke and tired. There are days I feel the burnout and wonder how much longer I can do this.

But when I lie in bed each night and think about my day, I know that I helped an animal and I helped a person or few. I know that my life is not a waste and I know that I'm not just taking up space in the world; I'm giving back to the environment in the only small way I can.

I look around me at the other great rehabbers; people that have done this longer than I have and still keep going despite medical problems and personal challenges. I know that wildlife rehab is their life. These dedicated people inspire me and I hope that we can inspire you.

Good luck and best wishes in whatever you choose to do with your life!

978-0-595-48334

0-595-48334-8

www.ingramcontent.com/pod-product-compliance
Lightning Source LLC
Chambersburg PA
CBHW030405290526
45785CB00004B/1910